JUST YOUR
TYPE

JUST YOUR
TYPE

The Ultimate Guide to Eating and Training Right for Your Body Type

BY PHIL CATUDAL

WITH STACEY COLINO

Da Capo

LIFE
LONG

Da Capo Press
Hachette Book Group
1290 Avenue of the Americas, New York, NY 10104
www.dacapopress.com
@DaCapoPress

Printed in the United States of America
First Edition: May 2019
Published by Da Capo Press, an imprint of Perseus Books, LLC, a subsidiary of Hachette Book Group, Inc.

The Hachette Speakers Bureau provides a wide range of authors for speaking events. To find out more, go to www.hachettespeakersbureau.com or call (866) 376-6591.
The publisher is not responsible for websites (or their content) that are not owned by the publisher.

Print book interior design by Linda Mark.

Library of Congress Cataloging-in-Publication Data
Names: Catudal, Phil, author. | Colino, Stacey, author.
Title: Just your type: the ultimate guide to eating and training right for your body type / by Phil Catudal with Stacey Colino.
Description: First edition. | New York: Da Capo Lifelong Books, 2019. |
Includes bibliographical references and index.
Identifiers: LCCN 2019003497| ISBN 9780738285481 (pbk.: alk. paper) | ISBN 9780738285474 (e-book)
Subjects: LCSH: Physical fitness. | Exercise. | Diet. | Somatotypes.
 Classification: LCC GV481 .C39 2019 | DDC 613.7—dc23
LC record available at https://lccn.loc.gov/2019003497
ISBNs: 978-0-7382-8548-1 (paperback); 978-0-7382-8547-4 (ebook)

LSC-C

10 9 8 7 6 5 4 3 2

To my angel mum and superhero dad: this is for you.

CONTENTS

INTRODUCTION

B E HONEST: AT THIS VERY MOMENT, DO YOU HAVE THE BODY you want? I'm guessing the answer is *no* since you've picked up this book. Well, you're in good company (and you definitely get props for coming clean about this). Many people discover that even after they've been killing it at the gym or sticking with a wholesome, balanced diet, they don't get the results they were hoping for in terms of changing their body shape or body composition. Maybe they can't shed the body fat or gain the muscle definition they've been striving for. Or maybe they don't get the energy or stamina they want. Or maybe they don't achieve the personal record they were working toward. This may be because while they appeared to be doing everything right, they were actually following the optimal protocol for someone else's body, not their own. In other words, it might have been the ideal approach for their best friend or boss but not for them.

At any given hour during the day, millions of Americans are working out—running, lifting weights, or engaging in some other form of cardiovascular or resistance training. For the first time ever, in 2016 more than half of people in the United States reported that they were getting the minimum amount of exercise recommended by health experts, according to the Centers for Disease Control and Prevention. While that's a major milestone, in my experience approximately 70 percent of people are exercising the wrong way for their bodies' needs. To put it another way, for every 10 people who are exercising or working out, only about 3 of them are doing what it takes for them to achieve results efficiently.

Confused? Here's the backstory: every single one of us has a genetic blueprint that dictates our body type (a.k.a. somatotype). Every body type has its advantages so don't judge. But different body types do respond differently to certain dietary regimens or fitness programs. So, if you haven't achieved the fitness or weight control results you've been aiming for, this may be because you weren't providing *your* body with the physical challenges or the nutrients it needed to transform its appearance and physical condition. It's not your fault since you probably didn't have the fitness know-how or the right tools to do this. So don't beat yourself up about what didn't go right in the past, and stop bemoaning the build you were born with. It's time to take a different tack.

Whether you have a naturally athletic or curvaceous build or a physique that's slender, wiry, or willowy, there's good news: with the right exercise modalities and the right foods, you can turn the body you have into the body you want, losing inches, dropping pounds, and developing a more sculpted look in the process. You can perform better at certain sports, gain energy and stamina, and improve your overall health along the way. The key is to work *with* your individual body, rather than against it, based on your natural somatotype. There are three basic body types—ectomorphs, mesomorphs, and endomorphs—that can determine how you respond to certain foods and physical activities, what your hormonal and metabolic characteristics are, and how much lean muscle and body fat you have (and where it's located). This is something else you can partially thank your parents for: research suggests that a person's somatotype is 56 to 68 percent inherited (for the record, the mesomorph type has the highest degree of heritability), according to researchers from York University in Canada. Few people are purebreds, though, as far as body types go; instead, most people have a mix of characteristics from different somatotypes.

Once you identify and understand what your body type is, you'll discover how to work with it to achieve your weight and fitness goals. Adjusting your diet, your objectives, and expectations and adapting your workout approach to suit your DNA-determined reality can help you get to that prize. In other words, you *can* cultivate what you didn't get automatically from your genetic makeup. There are limits, of course: eating more healthfully or training more efficiently for your body type won't make you taller or change your bone structure—but it can change your body composition, as well as the way you feel, for the better. And that's where this book comes in: you'll learn how to put together a diet and exercise plan that's designed for your natural-born body type so that you can fuel it optimally with your food choices and enhance it with the right workout approaches to achieve your goals to get fitter, stronger, sexier, and more self-assured.

Trust me on this because I'm personally and professionally familiar with the importance of working with your body, instead of against it. After winning a five-year battle against childhood leukemia (I was the bald kid in my kindergarten photo because of chemo), I became a fitness freak in my teens and developed a diet and exercise regimen that helped me become super strong and fit; before I knew it, people at the gym were begging me to train them. I thought about becoming a doctor but decided that instead of treating people who were sick, I wanted to help people avoid going down the path to disease or illness. Today, I am a highly successful global health coach and celebrity trainer based in Los Angeles and a father of three.

I have been training celebrities for more than 10 years, and I'm consistently able to give my clients results faster than they ever thought possible—even faster than other top trainers achieve with *their* clients. Just like our bodies aren't mirror images of each other, our exercise and dietary regimens shouldn't be carbon copies, either. That's why generic weight-loss or shape-up programs often don't work for the people who try them. To achieve success, you need to work *with* your natural body type and do the optimal combination of cardio, strength training, and flexibility exercises and consume the right proportion of carbohydrates, protein, and fats, also known as macronutrients, for *your* physique.

By the time you finish this book, you will be on your way to becoming your own personal trainer and dietitian. You'll have put yourself in the driver's seat, and you'll be steering yourself toward becoming the strongest, fittest, healthiest version of you yet. The ultimate goal is not to achieve anybody else's idea of the perfect body or stellar lifestyle; it's to translate your own get-fit, get-healthy goals and your good intentions into effective actions that will help you feel more powerful, more comfortable, and more vibrant in your own skin. That's a feel-good type everyone can relate to and achieve.

While fitness trends and fad diets will come and go, your body type is the one constant that's never going to change. The message behind *Just Your Type* is simple but powerful—if you want to be healthy, fit, slim, and strong, focus on the physical and dietary moves that will enhance your natural-born body type. This book is based on the successful training protocol that I use with my celebrity clients, and it will give you better results in weeks than you've had with months of training or dieting in the past. These impressive outcomes are possible because my program will give your body the fuel and physical challenges it needs, not the ones it doesn't. The workout that your willowy friend (an ectomorph) swears by isn't likely to give you the results you crave if you're strong and muscular (a mesomorph) or softer and more curvaceous (an endomorph). The right training approach and the right calories really do make all the difference. While the goal with my plan is to maximize your health and master your strength, weight loss (or body fat loss) is usually a positive side effect.

Stick with the sensible, targeted program in this book, and you'll not only get leaner and more energized, but also you'll emerge stronger, healthier, and looking and feeling the way you've been wanting to. There are no gimmicks or catches or torturous moves—I promise. This is the most effective diet and workout routine you'll ever follow, and you'll see results faster than you ever thought possible. Whatever body type you have, there is a diet and exercise formula that will provide you with an express ticket to a fabulous physique, improved health, and greater strength. Let's get started and find the one that's right for you.

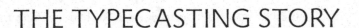

THE TYPECASTING STORY

WE LIVE IN A CULTURE THAT LOVES TO CATEGORIZE PEOPLE— by marital status, occupation, financial status, religion, recreational interests, personality types, zodiac signs, zip codes . . . you name it. Our bodies aren't much different, in this respect. As it happens, there are primary body types (somatotypes)— ectomorph, mesomorph, or endomorph—that each of us was naturally born with. One isn't better than the others are so there's no judgment here, and many of us tend to be a blend (or hybrid) of two different types. You could be a combination of a mesomorph and endomorph or an ectomorph and mesomorph, for example.

It's important to know your type because there's no one-size-fits-all diet and exercise regimen that will work for everyone.

That's why many people end up with a history of yo-yo dieting or going on and off various fitness fads—because they fail to get the results they thought they'd signed up for. So what worked for your friend may or may not work for you. By focusing on *your* somatotype, you can learn how to be more efficient in your training and how to fuel your body with the foods it will thrive on. Long story short: you can get a better body and be healthier faster by choosing the workouts and the right calories from the right sources that will work for your somatotype—and skip the ones that won't. Don't get me wrong: my version of sweat equity does take work and discipline. The difference with this plan is that you'll see and feel changes in your body more quickly than you ever have with other programs because this one is so efficient and effective.

Take a moment to think about this: Why would you take a slow, laborious route that may or may not give you the body of your dreams when there's a safe, efficient way for you to gain more lean muscle mass, develop a trimmer physique, and shed body fat two or three times faster than your current workout routine might allow, without subjecting yourself to excessive amounts of exercise or food deprivation? Choosing the laborious route would be like taking a three-stop flight from New York to California when a direct flight could get you to your destination in half the time and for the exact same price. It's a no-brainer and it really *is* that simple to transform your health and your body if you take the right approach, as I discovered firsthand.

As a teenager, I got into weightlifting, and while I gained significant strength pretty quickly, I couldn't attain the size or the defined musculature my older brother had, even when we did the same exercise regimen. Meanwhile, I got friends to come to the gym with me, and we soon discovered that even when we followed the same workout schedule, did the same exercises, the same reps and sets, the program produced completely different results for all of us. One friend's arms blew up into big, chiseled muscles (we were all jealous), while I was the guy with the lean "V taper" (broad, muscular shoulders with a tight waist), and another friend developed insanely strong legs and a six-pack. That's when I began researching body types and training needs—and found out that I'm a hybrid (an ecto-mesomorph) while my brother is a straight-up mesomorph, which explains a lot about why we responded so differently to the same workouts.

THE SKINNY ON BODY TYPES

As I learned in my research, the concept of somatotypes was developed in the 1940s when American psychologist and physician William Herbert Sheldon, M.D., Ph.D., sought to correlate body types with physical strengths and weaknesses, personality characteristics, and behavior. Over the years, there has been some controversy about somatotypes, partly because not that many people fit neatly into one of the three primary categories (more on that later) but also because the notion of "constitutional psychology," or personality attributes being related to specific body types, is pretty hard to swallow. There isn't a shred of evidence to suggest that someone's body type, composition, or shape determines his or her temperament, psychological makeup, or other personality attributes. So let me just say: IMO, those claims are utter nonsense. I know men and women who happen to be endomorphs or ectomorphs who are assertive and bold (traits traditionally attributed to mesomorphs); similarly, I know endomorphs or mesomorphs who are introverted and self-conscious (qualities linked with ectomorphs). You undoubtedly do, too. Different personalities come in a variety of body shapes and sizes, so let's agree to throw the personality part of the equation out of the picture without rejecting the whole somatotype concept.

After all, exercise scientists, physicians, and other health experts have seen great merit in studying significant differences in the physiques, hormonal responses, and physical performances between the somatotype profiles that Sheldon outlined. And there is solid science behind using somatotyping for fitness and athletic training to enhance performance. Of course, there are genetic, hormonal, anatomical, metabolic, digestive, and other variables in every individual that make that person's body different from others who have the same body type. But notwithstanding these differences, certain body types are a lot more alike than they are different.

I love what I do specifically because I like to find the optimal approach for every individual, to tailor a program that will work best for him or her—I consider myself a physique transformation specialist. The fact that I'm delivering consistent results speaks volumes for my approach, which is why I have embraced it both personally and professionally. In my 10-plus years as a professional in the health and fitness industry, I have yet to find a superior or more efficient and effective approach to helping clients, friends, and family members consistently achieve their health and fitness goals.

Consider my client, Ashley, 24, who had suffered from eating disorders and body dysmorphia (a condition involving obsessing over perceived flaws in your appearance) and felt demoralized because she didn't look like the models she would see on Instagram. At 5'6" and 140 pounds, Ashley was eating healthfully and exercising three hours a day—and she just couldn't understand how or why she didn't look like those models. After discussing how the media distorts reality in fashion pics (thanks to the use of filters, lighting, editing techniques, and the like), I explained the importance of setting realistic goals for her body type. I also told her that she was seriously over-exercising, and though her food choices were healthy, she was severely under-eating; as a result, she was spiking her levels of the stress hormone cortisol, which was reducing her metabolic efficiency and promoting fat storage. An almost pure mesomorph, Ashley's body was naturally strong and muscular, with broad shoulders and a compact torso. Many women would love to look like her! For her, the "problem" was that she wanted a long, lean midsection and to be 15 to 20 pounds lighter, with narrow hips.

Here's what we did: we took her workouts down from about 15 hours a week to 6, with three weight-training/high-intensity-interval workout days (focused on calisthenics and building strength) and three days of cardio work-outs, plus increasing her calorie intake in a controlled but significant manner. Within two weeks, she had lost three pounds and felt so much better. "But I'm eating more!" she said at one point. "I don't get it!" By 12 weeks in, she had dropped 8 pounds and looked leaner in the ways she wanted, with a slimmer waist and abdomen and shapely muscles. With the right training, she learned how to maximize her body's natural musculature and fat-burning efficiency— and ended up looking and feeling better than she'd ever felt before.

There are loads of success stories just like Ashley's. But let's get down to business with the basic 411 about body types. Here's a high-altitude look at how the different types compare:

- **Ectomorphs** tend to be lean and slender, with a small to medium frame and relatively long limbs. They typically have a fast metabolism, which is why they sometimes struggle to maintain their weight, and they tolerate a high-carbohydrate intake well. Ectomorphs' bodies are well suited to endurance sports (like long-distance running or cycling), though they're somewhat prone to lower back and knee injuries; they have a hard time adding or maintaining muscle mass. (Famous examples: supermodel Gisele, former president Barack Obama, tennis great Roger Federer, Olympic gold medalist swimmer Michael Phelps, and actors Brad Pitt and Cameron Diaz.)
- **Mesomorphs** usually have a medium bone structure, with broad shoulders, a relatively small waist, and a naturally muscular, athletic build even without working out. If they're physically active, they tend to add and maintain strength and lean muscle mass easily (even when they have breaks in training). Their metabolisms are efficient, they tolerate carbohydrates well (thanks to their body's efficient insulin response), and they can lose body fat relatively easily. (Celebrity examples: actors Jennifer Garner, Angela Bassett, Mark Wahlberg, and Dwayne "The Rock" Johnson;

pop superstar Madonna; tennis champ Serena Williams; and actor/former
California governor Arnold Schwarzenegger.)

✦ **Endomorphs** generally have a larger bone structure with wider hips,
more narrow shoulders, and more pear-shaped bodies with higher
amounts of body fat. Compared to the other types, their metabolisms
are slower, they tend to gain weight easily, and they're very sensitive to
carbohydrates because they often have insulin resistance challenges. As
a result, they often respond better to diets that are high in protein and
very low in carbs. Endomorphs tend to lose body fat slowly but they
have an easier time building muscle than ectomorphs do. (For examples,
visualize pop superstars Jennifer Lopez and Beyoncé, actors Sofía Vergara, Chris Pratt, and Russell Crowe, and late-night TV talk show host
James Corden.)

As previously mentioned, few people are 100 percent ectomorph, endomorph, or mesomorph (and btw, you'll learn much more about these types
in the chapters to come). Most people are hybrids with combinations of the
various qualities associated with different body types. The most common natural hybrids are ecto-mesomorphs (with long, lean limbs and a broad chest
and shoulders and endo-mesomorphs (who have wide, thick, but compact
physiques that are muscular, not soft). In addition, there are people who are
endo-ectomorphs (with thin legs but substantial fat storage in the midsection).
More often than not, these folks have developed this body type as a result of
their behavior, not genetics—maybe they started out as ectomorphs but then
gained some endomorph qualities, thanks to years of consuming poor-quality
diets and sticking with sedentary habits. It's not an innate body type but it's
fairly common in the modern world.

Somatotypes clearly have a genetic component. If you look at photos of
your parents' physiques when they were between the ages of 15 and 25 then
look at your own body, you'll likely see that your body type resembles one or

the other of them or maybe a mix of both. Though it's possible for individuals to carry a recessive gene, it's unusual for two endomorphs to spawn an ectomorph or for two ectomorphs to create a mesomorph. Sure, you can be a hybrid body type, but you'll likely have more dominant body traits from your parents, with fewer variations that are unique to you. But that doesn't mean that your DNA-determined somatotype is your destiny. A natural-born endomorph can certainly do what it takes to get lean, while ectomorphs can corrupt their bodies (with bad food and no exercise) and become overweight. The human body is an amazingly adaptable organism and it can be transformed in significant ways, good or bad. The key questions are, *How well or badly will you treat yours?* And, *How badly do you want to change your physique?*

GIVING YOUR BODY WHAT IT NEEDS

The truth is, each type (and hybrid) has its inherent perks and pitfalls, but you can take effective steps to work with your natural-born body type and achieve a new personal best. You may not always realize it but your body really is on your side and it can deliver the results you're seeking—but only if *you're* on your body's side. In other words, you need to consider: Are you giving your body what *it* needs to achieve the results you're seeking? Chances are, the answer is (1) No; or (2) I'm not really sure. (Otherwise, you wouldn't have picked up this book.)

With the right approach, each type and every hybrid can be trained into optimal shape and better health. With the wrong approach, well, not so much. Some people will lose more weight by eating a higher percentage of healthy fats, while others will respond better to high-carb or high-protein plans. For example, while a high-carb diet will work fine for ectomorphs, it won't help endomorphs who might end up gaining weight even if they have a lower overall calorie intake. By contrast, a low-carb, high-fat approach (like the ketogenic diet) won't help ectomorphs, who could end up losing muscle mass and feeling intensely tired on the plan. (Spoiler alert: mesomorphs have it easiest when it comes to diet.)

Your body type also can affect the way you respond to exercise. In a study involving men between the ages of 18 and 40 with different dominant body types, researchers from the USDA found that while all the groups had the same peak power output, the ectomorphs had the greatest respiratory exchange ratio (which affects their muscles' capacity to get energy) during peak aerobic exercise and the greatest blood lactate concentrations after exercise (a sign of greater fatigue). A study from Tunisia found that after participating in a 12-week program consisting of two aerobic-endurance training sessions per week, adults with mesomorph or meso-endomorph body types showed the greatest improvements in their aerobic capacity.

Meanwhile, various studies have tried to establish a link between certain somatotypes and performance in particular sports. For example, in a 2015 study, researchers examined the somatotypes among high-profile Lithuanian athletes in kayaking, basketball, and soccer and found some interesting differences: elite kayakers and basketball players tended to have endomorphic bodies while the high-profile soccer players had ectomorphic types. By contrast, a 2014 study examined the influence of somatotypes on success in sport climbing among men and found that the endomorphic attributes had a significant influence on their success. In another 2014 study, researchers from Spain analyzed the body type characteristics of elite female volleyball players from the highest Spanish league and found that mesomorphs dominated. A 2018 study from Spain found that while female Olympic race walkers tend to be endomorphs, male Olympic race walkers are more likely to be mesomorphs. And a 2017 study found that world and Olympic mountain bike champions typically have ecto-mesomorphic bodies.

All of this goes to show that people with different body types can excel at a variety of sports. But you also have to consider the possibility that "like attracts like"—that because people expect those with very tall, lean frames to be good at basketball, they might naturally gravitate toward playing hoops if they have that kind of physique. That slender people with long, lanky limbs might be natural-born runners. Or, that if you have a naturally muscular, athletic build, you might be good at football or bodybuilding. Similarly, if a girl has a petite, compact body, she might see herself fitting in among gymnasts. The point is, people may think they belong in a certain sport because they look like the other players or athletes, so they pursue it, train for it, and excel in it. In other words, there may be a natural selection process at play here.

While you might indeed excel at certain sports or athletic activities because of your body type or your natural physical prowess, you are certainly not limited by your body characteristics. There doesn't have to be a sports-oriented destiny for your body type—I promise. Regardless of your somatotype, you can train to get your body into peak shape so you'll have a fair chance to perform at your best in the activity of your choice—but only if you do the right training for your body type. The key is to optimize your training for your body type and the activity you want to pursue or the goal you want to achieve.

Whether your aim is to shed excess body fat or build muscle, knowing your body type can help you maximize your results. The right training approach and the right calories really do make all the difference. Working harder isn't always the answer but working *smarter* is. People are creatures of habit and tend to do things the same way consistently, including the same cardio or strength-building workouts or using the same bad form that compromises their results. It's a bit like driving a convertible in chilly weather with the top down and the heat on—operating at cross-purposes with your goal. Take my client Steve Howey (who plays Kevin on *Shameless*) as an example: He's 6'4", and when we started working together, he weighed 240 pounds. He had been training and eating like an ectomorph when he's really an endo-mesomorph hybrid. In short, he was eating too many carbs and doing a classic bodybuilding program for lean, skinny guys who want to pack on muscle. While Steve was doing the right exercises, he wasn't doing them in the right order or tempo or performing the right combo of reps and sets. With some tweaks to his training and eating regimen, he was able to drop 25 pounds of body fat and add 10 pounds of lean muscle (he now weighs 215 pounds); he also gained a six-pack on his abs and has become one of the fittest, most muscular Hollywood stars today. The kicker: he is now doing triathlons!

The reality is, very few people see themselves accurately, and in my experience, about 50 percent misclassify their body type: endomorphs may think they're mesomorphs, or ectomorphs may identify themselves as endomorphs, especially if they have a soft midsection. In the next chapter, you'll learn how to accurately identify your true type with a quiz—it's the crucial first step in creating an individualized workout and diet plan that's tailored to *your* body shape and composition.

By pinpointing and learning about your body type, you'll be on your way to becoming your own personal trainer and nutritionist. You'll become more attuned to how your body responds to certain foods in terms of your energy levels, your mental clarity, your digestion, and sleep quality. You'll learn why certain exercise regimens will work for you but maybe not for your friends or workout buddies. Along the way, you'll naturally improve your quality of life and sense of well-being. *Are you ready?* The ball is in your court and in your hands, and you've got a clear path to the basket . . . See it. Feel it. It's time for you to drive, soar, and nail that slam dunk!

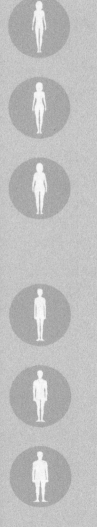

WHAT'S *YOUR* BODY TYPE?

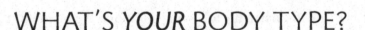

IF YOU'RE LIKE MANY PEOPLE, YOU MIGHT ANSWER THIS QUESTION
with a response like "hot," "weak," "strong," "flabby," "curvy,"
or another adjective. In your defense, trying to evaluate your
own body type in the abstract is a loaded proposition because
there's a good chance you're judging it based on what you wish it
looked like, rather than how it actually looks right now. But there
are ways to ditch the subjective judgments and figure out what
your natural-born body type is, objectively speaking. If you were
to talk to your doctor about your weight and body type, the conversation would inevitably gravitate toward Body Mass Index
(BMI), which indicates if you are underweight, normal weight,
overweight, or obese. In my opinion, BMI is a vague, outdated

measurement because it doesn't account for your body composition—variables such as muscle, water, fat, hormones, or bone size, all of which are important. Based on the BMI charts, I fall somewhere between the overweight and obese categories, but my excess weight is all muscle (I have 9.5 percent body fat). Healthcare professionals use BMI because it's the only standardized way to compare people's bodies and create some sort of database regarding a person's height-to-weight ratio.

To get a more precise assessment of your body composition, you could go to a lab and have your body fat, bone, and muscle mass measured, then have various ratios calculated, which would give you a scientific result. But there's an easier, more accessible (and less expensive) way to gauge your body type at home. And I'm about to walk you through it. So grab something to write with and let's get to it.

Read each of the following questions or statements thoroughly and choose the option that best describes you. Be honest in your responses (you won't be graded on this!). If you're not sure which of two responses applies to you, trust your instincts or choose both (you'll see why later).

1. From an objective point of view, which of the following issues seems most prominent (or dominant) on your body when you look in the mirror?
   a. Bone
   b. Muscle
   c. Body fat
2. How do your shoulders compare to your hips?
   a. My shoulders are narrower than my hips.
   b. They're approximately the same width as my hips.
   c. My shoulders are wider than my hips.
3. Which of the following objects best describes your body shape?
   a. A pencil

   b. An hourglass

   c. A pear

4. If you encircle one wrist with your other hand's middle finger and thumb, what happens?

   a. My middle finger and thumb overlap a bit.

   b. My middle finger and thumb touch, but just barely.

   c. There's a gap between my middle finger and thumb.

5. When it comes to your weight, which of the following patterns best describes your history?

   a. I have trouble gaining muscle weight or body fat.

   b. I can gain and lose weight without too much difficulty.

   c. I gain weight easily but have a hard time losing it.

6. Think about what your body looked like, before you corrupted it with poor dietary and exercise habits, once you reached your full height as a teenager or young adult. How did you look?

   a. I looked long and lanky.

   b. I looked strong and compact.

   c. I looked soft and full bodied.

7. If you'd been exercising regularly and you were to take a break for a few months, what would happen to your body?

   a. I would lose muscle and strength quickly.

   b. My body wouldn't change that much.

   c. My body would soften up significantly and I might even gain weight.

8. Put on a pair of form-fitting jeans—where on your body do they get extra clingy or even stuck?

   a. They don't. In fact, I can't keep them up without a belt.

   b. With a bit of work, I can wriggle my way into them over my muscular thighs.

   c. They get caught on my butt or belly.

9. When you have a serious carb-fest (think: heaping plate of pasta or multiple slices of pizza), how do you feel afterward?

   a. The same as I usually do—normal, really.

   b. I generally feel good, though I notice my ab muscles are extra hard or my belly feels full.

   c. More often than not, I feel tired or bloated for a few hours after the meal.

10. How would you describe your body's bone structure?

   a. I have a small frame.

   b. I have a medium frame.

   c. I have a relatively large frame.

TIME FOR SCORING

Add up the number of times you answered A, B, or C. If you chose mostly A's, you're an ectomorph; mostly B's, you're a mesomorph; mostly C's, you're an endomorph. If your responses were divided fairly equally—as in 5 and 5 or even 6 and 4—between two different letters, you likely have a hybrid body type. To be specific, if your responses were split between A's and B's, you're an ecto-mesomorph; if they're spread between B's and C's, you're a meso-endomorph; and if you found your responses in a 50–50 or 60–40 split between A's and C's, you're an ecto-endomorph. If you end up with a 7–3 division between two different types, it may mean that you've strayed off course from your true type with poor dietary choices, in which case the hybrid approach will steer you back on the right track.

Here's what this form of typecasting really says about you:

ECTOMORPHS: Generally thin and lean, ectomorphs tend to have slender waists, narrow hips and shoulders, small joints, and long legs and arms. They tend to be slim, without much body fat or noticeable muscle mass. Because

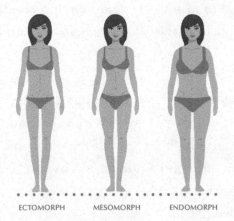

ECTOMORPH   MESOMORPH   ENDOMORPH

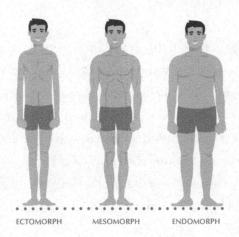

ECTOMORPH   MESOMORPH   ENDOMORPH

they have fast metabolisms, they burn calories quickly, so ectomorphs may find themselves hungry frequently throughout the day; yet, regardless of what, how often, or how much they eat, they don't gain weight or muscle easily.

MESOMORPHS: Naturally muscular, mesomorphs typically have moderate-size frames, with wider shoulders and a narrow waist, strong arms and legs, and modest amounts of body fat. They are genetically predisposed to build muscle so mesomorphs often require a slightly higher calorie intake (since muscle requires more calories to maintain it) and more protein than the other types do (again, for muscle maintenance). Generally, mesomorphs are able to lose or gain weight easily.

ENDOMORPHS: Because they have a medium-to-large bone structure and more body fat than the other types, women who are endomorphs are often described as curvaceous or full-figured, while endomorphic men might be considered stocky, doughy, or round. Endomorphs usually have narrow shoulders and wider hips and carry any excess weight in the lower abdomen, hips, and thighs. It's often challenging for them to lose weight but with the right diet and training approach, it can be done.

ECTO-MESOMORPHS: These hybrids are increasingly common, especially in the athletic world where this physique is prized for being aesthetically appealing. In fact, for men and women alike, ecto-mesomorphs tend to have the "fitness model" look. Often muscular with V-shaped torsos (think: wide upper back, developed chest and shoulders, narrow waist), ecto-mesomorphs are lean and agile, with strong-looking (but not bulky) arms and legs. (Btw: I'm an ecto-mesomorph. I've always been naturally long and lean, and I was able to build significant muscle with the right diet and exercise regimen.)

MESO-ENDOMORPHS: Including variations where people have more predominantly mesomorphic or endomorphic qualities (rather than a truly even split), this is the most common hybrid, according to research. Many bodybuilders and contact sports athletes (like football players) have this body type. Characterized by thick arms and legs and a boxy chest and mid-section, this type looks powerful but it isn't chiseled. (This may be partly because people with this body type tend to retain water and a layer of fat on top of their muscles.) People with this kind of build who want to get a leaner physique should be prepared to take a more refined approach to resistance training, cardio work-outs, and diet, so they can prioritize fat loss.

ECTO-ENDOMORPHS: Usually, this is a behaviorally acquired body type—basically, someone who is really an ectomorph has added significant body fat, whether it's from poor eating habits, sedentary ways, or a combo of these less-than-stellar habits. With long limbs and a smaller bone structure, ecto-endomorphs often have soft midsections, droopy chests, and flabby upper arms and legs from sheer neglect. To improve fitness, body composition, and health, the most efficient plan for this type involves resistance training and high-intensity cardio, both of which promote muscle growth and stimulate metabolism. Since ecto-endomorphs may have developed some insulin resistance, their bodies may not be as efficient at burning carbohydrates so I recommend a dietary plan that's suited to endomorphs—with a slightly higher protein intake, a medium fat intake, and lower carb levels—until the excess body fat comes off and metabolic function is optimized; then, these hybrid types can switch to more of an ectomorph approach (adding in more carbs).

WHAT ALL THIS MEANS FOR YOU

Now that you have a greater understanding of your body type, you're in a better position to alter your diet and fitness regimens to suit your body's needs. Remember: generally, body types lie on a spectrum, rather than being distinct points on a grid or graph. Chances are, you have either a dominant body type with characteristics of another one or a true combination body type that's evenly split between two different ones. Already, this increased awareness and knowledge probably put you a few steps ahead of where you were. If you're like many people, you've probably misjudged your body type in the past, whether it was because you didn't understand the different somatotypes, you had general body insecurities, or you were excessively critical about your body. Let's face it: it's a common phenomenon. In my experience, about 50 percent of people get their body type wrong, and the media and social media can lead any of us to compare our bodies to unrealistic standards and come up with skewed perceptions of our own physiques. But remember: the body ideals portrayed in the media are often digitally altered or enhanced with special filters, lighting, or other forms of manipulation, which means they're not natural or real. Which means you've been comparing yourself to an illusion, really. Alternatively, you might misclassify your body type based on comments your parents or other influential adults made to you over the years or phantom body-image issues you have now (if you used to be heavier or had an eating disorder, for example). It could be that you're discounting the proportion of muscle you have on your body and erroneously equating size with body fat, or that you have a mental health condition such as body dysmorphia (an obsessive focus on a perceived flaw in your appearance). Whatever is at the root of your past body misclassification, it could mean that you've been training the wrong way because you've been viewing and treating your body the wrong way.

Or, maybe you had an accurate sense of what your body type is but you jumped on the latest fitness fad or diet du jour, regardless of whether it was appropriate for your physique. The problem is, that's like trying to rebuild or maintain your car's engine using the wrong manual (such as the one from your motorboat or moped). At best, it's ineffective and a waste of time; at worst, it can bite you in the a**.

I've met plenty of people who know they're endomorphs but they defiantly believe they can out-exercise their lousy diets and their body's natural physiology. Or, they concentrate on crash diets and cardio workouts and end up eating too little, restricting their calories and carbohydrates excessively and continuously riding the yo-yo-diet rollercoaster with peaks, valleys, and binges along the way; meanwhile, they're surprised when they don't end up building muscle definition or reaching their long-term fitness goals.

Similarly, there are ectomorphs out there who have slipped into the ecto-endo zone over time and come to perceive themselves as pure endomorphs because of the excess pounds they've added to their frames (essentially they've become "skinny-fat" with slim arms and legs and a rounder midsection). At the gym, some of them will spend 45 minutes a day on the treadmill or the elliptical; they might restrict their carb intake and avoid eating anything after 6 p.m.—and still be unable to transform their physiques the way they want to. What they should be doing is ditching the immediate gratification of cardio-intensive, calorie-burning workouts and focusing on the big picture instead: adding lean muscle mass to their physiques through the right pattern of resistance training and following the optimal dietary plan (with enough calories) to fuel their muscles and their metabolism, as you'll see in the chapters that follow.

GETTING AND KEEPING IT REAL

When I start working with a new client, the first step is usually for us to get to know each other in person, usually over coffee, outside of the gym. I like to get a sense of what clients' lives are like at work and home, how high their stress levels are, what their eating and exercise habits are like, what their weight history is, and what their current fitness goals are. This way, I can get a sense of what real-world challenges might end up creating roadblocks or ultimately derailing their best intentions. In other words, I'm trying to gauge what's realistic for us to do in an efficient manner. After all, most people can't completely reorganize their lives to make body transformation their top priority, nor do they have the financial resources to hire the trainers, nutritionists, personal chefs, and other assistants who can support the cause (the way many Hollywood people do).

Hot tip: if you've been using a particular diet or workout approach for a month and nothing about your body has changed, it's not right for you. It's that simple. Let's say a client tells me she gets bloated after eating certain foods (such as dairy products, items with lots of sugar or refined flour, fried foods, and other pro-inflammatory foods) or another client shows me his "soft" body and says he eats 100 percent vegan and has been doing body-weight workouts three times per week to try to gain muscle definition and tightness to no avail. Between hearing either history and doing a quick visual assessment of the person, I would probably have an "aha" moment—realizing that she or he is a pure ectomorph, in which case the approach the person was taking wouldn't deliver the desired results for her or his body type.

With the right approach, can I help you look like Henry Cavill in *Superman* or Gal Gadot in *Wonder Woman?* Sure, but it will take a heckuva lot of hard work and discipline so it's important to get a reality check about what you are willing to do to reach your goals before moving forward. The truth is, consistency trumps nearly everything else when it comes to body transformation, which is why it's essential to figure out what's realistic for you to commit to; that way, I can develop a workout and meal plan that make sense for you and your life.

Part of this assessment process involves evaluating a client's body type. After training people for so many years, I often have an instinct for what a person's natural body type is, but as we all know, looks can be deceiving. And sometimes my initial hunches may be off base, especially if the person has significantly changed his or her body through dieting, exercise, or even surgery.

Since you and I can't meet for coffee (though I wish we could), it's up to you to gauge *your* body type so that you can then choose the approach that seems to best suit your physique's natural tendencies and your personal goals. My aim with this book is to help you become your own personal trainer and nutritionist. So take yourself out for coffee, think about what your life is like at work and home, how high your stress level is, what your past weight history has been (it can help to look at old photos), and consider what your current goals are. Next, think about how hard you're willing to work to reach them, then go home and map out a plan of action.

When I first bring a client into the gym, I'll take body measurements—weight, height, and body fat percentage, as well as measuring his or her chest, waist, thigh, and arm circumference. Since I can't do this for you personally, enlist a friend or partner's help or go ahead and DIY (but keep in mind: having someone help you really does improve accuracy). Don't be scared away from doing this—it provides a baseline assessment of where you are now so you can track your progress. Taking measurements is an especially good way to do it because losing inches arguably counts more than the number on the scale (especially since muscle weighs more than body fat does but it looks tighter, more compact, and, well, just better).

You'll want to take four main measurements: around mid-biceps in your upper arms, at the thickest part of your upper thighs, around your bust/chest (at the fullest part), and around your natural waist (the narrowest part of your torso between your belly button and your breastbone). It's essential to measure yourself correctly or you'll get a distorted sense of what's happening with your body; in other words, your measurements are only as accurate as your technique. So don't pull the tape too tightly or let it dig into your skin; also, don't flex your muscles, suck in your gut, or hold your breath while taking your measurements. Hold the tape straight and flat as you wrap it around each body part. Write down your measurements (in inches or centimeters, your choice) or keep a log on your smartphone and retake them every couple of weeks to gauge your progress. Trust me, numbers don't lie, so this is a great way to monitor your progress.

Whether you want to slim down or simply add definition to your muscles, the underlying goal is to harden your body, which means the numbers will generally shrink as you embark on the body-type program that's best for you. This means you'll be losing body fat and gaining lean muscle mass, which is probably just what you want. Even better, adding muscle mass to your frame through resistance training, which you'll do in some fashion with each of the body-type regimens, will increase the efficiency of your hormones (including testosterone, thyroid hormone, and growth hormone) as well as the function of your endocrine system (including insulin production and sensitivity and blood sugar regulation). What's more, your metabolic rate will pick up its pace once you have more muscle on your body, which means you won't have to sweat your calorie intake as much as you may have in the past.

Sounds promising, right? Let's get started! In the chapters that follow, you'll discover the best workout and dietary approaches for *your* body type, strategies that will help you achieve your long-term slim-down, get-toned, or shape-up goals. This will help you create a roadmap that will bring you to a destination where you'll feel and look fitter and function better than ever—and be able to sustain those benefits. Along the way, you'll come to understand the perks and challenges that are unique to your body type and figure out how to refine some of the nutrition and exercise aspects of your program so they're more effective for your body and your life. In that sense, this approach will become truly personalized—as in, just right for *your* type.

NEED-TO-KNOW BODY BASICS

W ITH THE STRATEGIC USE OF PHYSICAL AND DIETARY MOVES that will enhance your natural body type, you can become healthier, leaner, fitter, stronger, slimmer, more energized, and more self-assured than ever before. The right training approach and the right calories really do make all the difference. While the goal with the plans that follow is to maximize your health and master your strength, weight loss (or body fat loss) is usually a positive side effect. This means you really can turn the body you have into the body you want, losing inches, torching body fat, and developing a stronger, more sculpted look in the process.

To get to those goals, you need to work *with* your natural-born body type and do the optimal combination of cardio and strength-training exercises while consuming the right proportion of macro-nutrients for *your* physique. You'll learn how to do that in the chapters that follow. But before we get to the specific body-type plans, there are some basic body principles you should be familiar with because they apply to *every* body. No exceptions.

Let's start with metabolism, which is a series of biochemical reactions in your body that allows you to convert the calories from the food you eat into energy that your body can use. Everyone has a different resting or basal metabolic rate—the number of calories your body burns just to sustain basic functions like your heartbeat and breathing—and it's determined by several factors, including your gender (spoiler alert: men have the advantage), age (younger people have speedier metabolisms), your body composition (muscle wins over fat), and genetic factors. Even if some of these factors are working against you, by using the following plans you can optimize your metabolism by adjusting your diet, workout regimen, and lifestyle habits.

METABOLISM MATH

To get a pulse on where you are now, metabolically speaking, you can use the following formulas to assess approximately how many calories you burn each day. Note: you'll need to have handy your weight in kilograms (divide your weight in pounds by 2.2) and your height in centimeters (multiply your height in inches by 2.54), plus, your age in years.

IF YOU'RE A MAN: Multiply your body weight (in kg) times 10; next, multiply your height (in cm) by 6.25; add these two figures together and put it aside (consider this figure A). Now, multiply your age by 5 (consider this figure B). Subtract figure B from figure A, then add 5 to that sum to get your basal metabolic rate (BMR), the number of calories your body burns just to exist and fulfill the basic functions that keep you alive.

IF YOU'RE A WOMAN: Multiply your body weight (in kg) times 10; next, multiply your height (in cm) by 6.25; add these two figures together and put it aside (consider this sum figure A). Now, multiply your age by 5 (consider this figure B). Subtract figure B from figure A, then subtract 161 from that sum to get your basal metabolic rate (BMR).

Men   BMR = (10 × weight in kg) + (6.25 × height in cm) – (5 × age in years) + 5

Women   BMR = (10 × weight in kg) + (6.25 × height in cm) – (5 × age in years) – 161

Now, it's time to fine-tune that calculation, based on your level of physical activity. This will give you your body's total daily energy expenditure (TDEE, for short), the number of calories you burn in a day.

- If you are sedentary (meaning, you get little to no exercise), multiply your BMR by 1.2.
- If you are lightly active (meaning, you do light exercise or play sports for an hour a day, one to three times per week), multiply your BMR by 1.375.
- If you are moderately active (you exercise at a moderate intensity or play sports three to five days per week), multiply your BMR by 1.55.
- If you are very active (meaning, you go hard then go home for at least an hour at a time, six or seven days per week), multiply your BMR by 1.725.
- If you are extra active (if you do intense training every day for a competitive event, for example, or have a physically demanding job), multiply your BMR by 1.9.

To make these figures less abstract, consider a guy named Jesse, 38, who is 5'10" and weighs 190 pounds and is lightly active (say, he plays tennis two or three times per week). His BMR = (10 x 86.4) + (6.25 x 177.8) - (5 x 38) + 5, or 864 + 1,111.25 - 190 + 5 = 1,790.25. His TDEE is 1,790 x 1.375 or 2,461. That's how many calories he typically burns in a day.

If Jesse were a woman with the same height, weight, age, and physical activity level, her BMR would equal 1,624.25 and her TDEE would be 2,233 calories.

THERE ARE SEVERAL VARIABLES THAT CAN AFFECT YOUR METABOLIC RATE, including your body composition (how much lean muscle mass you have, compared to body fat), your conditioning level, and genetic factors. Pound for pound, muscle is more dense than body fat—and it requires more calories to maintain it. In fact, each pound of muscle you have uses 6 to 8 calories a day just to sustain itself, whereas every pound of fat requires only 2 calories daily. This means that if you have a higher percentage of body fat, you'll burn fewer calories at rest than a friend who is the same height, weight, and gender but has a higher percentage of muscle mass. The good news is, this also means that if you shed body fat and add lean muscle mass to your body, you'll naturally increase your body's resting metabolic rate 24/7.

An important note: I don't usually ask my clients (and I won't be asking you) to count calories. Doing so is tedious and people can easily become obsessed. That's not what we want here. If you stick with the macronutrient ranges and food serving sizes that are recommended in each plan, the calories will basically take care of themselves. But sometimes people like to know how many calories their bodies expend on a daily basis, which is why I've provided this information here. File it away under "interesting 411" for now. If you need to tweak your calorie intake later—because you find that you're losing or gaining weight too fast on the plan—then you can revisit the calorie issue and fine-tune your approach. (In these situations a good first step is to adjust your food intake up or down by 10 to 20 percent, depending on whether you're dropping or adding pounds too fast.)

NUTRITION KNOW-HOW

What you eat provides the energy for almost everything your body does, as well as fuel for your workouts and the building blocks for your body's post-exercise recovery. Using nutritious foods as sources of fuel, energy, and vitality will help you build lean, sculpted muscle and a healthy, resilient physique. Of course, your diet also affects whether you will gain weight, lose weight, or maintain your current weight. The adage that "calories in versus calories out" is often debated or disputed, but it really does matter in the weight-management equation. To lose weight, you need to consume fewer calories than you burn through everyday activities and your workouts. Create a deficit of 3,500 calories per week, and you can theoretically lose a pound a week.

But it's also more complicated than that. You've undoubtedly heard some people say "a calorie is a calorie." Well, it's not entirely true unless you're doing a laboratory experiment. In that case, 100 calories from a cookie will actually release the same amount of energy as 100 calories' worth of avocado. But that's not how different sources of calories work inside your body. Depending on what's in them, different foods have variable effects on your hunger, satiety, metabolism, digestion, energy, blood sugar levels, and fat storage.

So let's shift gears and talk a little about calories and where they come from. There are three classes of macronutrients—carbohydrates, protein, and fats—that together contribute to a healthy diet. While 1 gram of carbohydrates and 1 gram of protein each contains 4 calories, a gram of fat contains 9 calories—more than twice as many. But good fats do have a place in a healthy diet.

Let's take a closer look at these key players.

CARBOHYDRATES often get a bad rap in our culture but they are vital to life, contributing much of the energy you need for exercise and other physical activities as well as the functioning of your organs. But not all carbs are equal, so the source really does matter. Simple carbs (found in table sugar, sugary packaged foods, and refined starches) don't offer much in the way of nutrition and they lead to quick spikes (followed by crashes) in blood sugar levels; they also promote sneaky, internal inflammation that can harm your health. That's why added sugars and refined starches should be put on the no-fly list (not in your mouth).

By contrast, complex carbohydrates (found in vegetables, legumes, whole grains, nuts, and seeds) provide steadier, longer-lasting energy and greater nutritional value. Complex carbs are also high in fiber, which slows digestion, takes up a fair amount of space in the stomach, enhances feelings of fullness, and lowers blood sugar and insulin levels. Some body types are more efficient than others are at breaking down carbs (hello, ectomorphs!), so the proportion of carbs in the diet that's right for you depends partly on your body type, as you'll see.

PROTEIN provides the greatest and longest-lasting feeling of fullness, partly because it takes our bodies longer to digest protein than it does other macronutrients. Whenever you eat something, you gain a metabolic boost from digesting, processing, and storing food, a process that causes your body to generate heat, which helps it burn calories faster (this is called the thermic effect of eating). An added perk: eating protein means you end up burning calories for longer during the digestive process by stoking the metabolic furnace. With protein, too, quality counts so it's best to opt for fish and seafood, lean poultry or meats, eggs, nuts, and seeds. Getting enough protein in your diet is critical for building and maintaining muscle mass, repairing various tissues in the body, and providing a secondary source of energy for your body (carbohydrates are the main source).

FAT is often viewed as a dietary villain, but the human body needs healthy dietary fats to fulfill a variety of functions, including making hormones and cell membranes, aiding digestion and brain function, and promoting the absorption of fat-soluble vitamins. Sorry to be repetitive but . . . all dietary fat isn't created equal. Healthy fats include monounsaturated fats (in olive and peanut oils, most nuts and seeds, and avocado) and polyunsaturated fats (from omega-3 fatty acids and vegetable oils like sunflower and saf-flower oils). By contrast, consuming saturated fats (in fatty meats and full-fat dairy products) or trans fats (in many baked goods, snack foods, and fried foods—the word "hydrogenated" is a tip-off) increases hidden inflamma-tion throughout the body. So, avoid these as much as possible. (When it comes to saturated fats, make an exception for coconut oil, which contains medium-chain triglycerides that can be used as energy like carbohydrates; plus, it's been shown to reduce inflammation and help with overall hormone balance.)

Though it's not a macronutrient, water is an essential part of a healthy diet. For one thing, water is the most abundant substance in the body, ac-counting for about 60 percent of an adult's body weight, and since our bodies have no way to store water, we need to constantly replenish the fluids we lose through sweating, breathing, and performing other bodily functions. Accord-ing to the latest recommendations from the National Academies of Sciences, Engineering, and Medicine, an adequate daily fluid intake is about 15½ cups for men and 11½ cups for women (keep in mind that this includes fluids you get from foods, too). On each of the body-type plans, I recommend having 80 percent of your fluid intake come from water or seltzer and the rest can be from black coffee, green tea, or another type of tea. If you get bored with plain H_2O, you can add lemon wedges or cucumber slices. And if you can't stand black coffee, it's okay to add a little almond, cashew, or coconut milk (but not more than two or three times per day). Skip the juices, sodas, and alcohol. And it's best if you can steer clear of diet soda because there's some evidence that the artificial sweeteners they contain (especially sucralose) can actually ramp up your appetite. That's not what you want.

YOUR HORMONES AND YOUR HUNGER

IT'S NOT ONLY the insulin and blood sugar ups and downs that can affect your energy and eating habits throughout the day. With all body types, the ratio of the hormones ghrelin and leptin a person has can regulate his or her eating patterns. In a nutshell, ghrelin tells the brain that it's time to eat, thereby stimulating appetite, whereas leptin signals fullness or satiety in the brain—and turns on the body's fat-burning mechanism.

Unfortunately, some people can be leptin resistant, which means that while they're eating their brains send less of the "that's enough!" signals. If the ghrelin-leptin ratio is off, due to leptin resistance, the person's body is continuously telling his or her brain to "eat more!" without ever getting enough of the "stop eating!" signal. Not surprisingly, leptin resistance is more common among obese people.

Research shows that when people with leptin resistance or low leptin levels are given doses of leptin, they are able to recover normal metabolic and endocrine function. Who knows? Maybe some day, it will be routine to test people's ghrelin and leptin levels and supplement those that are out of whack. Until that happens, the onus is on you to do whatever you can to improve your body's hunger and satiety signals by optimizing your dietary choices, sleep habits, and other aspects of your lifestyle.

To become the fittest, healthiest version of you, it's important to stick with wholesome, nutritious, minimally processed foods. They'll help you naturally boost your energy and immune function, help you build and maintain lean muscle mass, and promote better digestion and brain function. When it comes to the body transformation process, consistency is key. It's true when it comes to your eating habits and your workouts. So eat regular meals and snacks to fuel your body properly. Don't skip meals or play the how-low-can-you-go game with calories. And don't forget to drink plenty of noncaffeinated fluids throughout the day. Your body needs a sufficient water intake to keep your metabolism humming and burning calories efficiently. So drink up with every meal and snack, as well as in between, and make sure you're well hydrated before, during, and after your workouts.

· · ·

PROTEIN PRODUCT PREFERENCES

IN THE BODY-TYPE plans that follow, you'll see that I recommend protein shakes and protein bars. Don't be fooled: while there are lots of different brands on the market, some of them are higher in protein than others. The ones that are higher in protein are the ones you want.

The protein powders I really like for protein shakes include Vega, which is a plant-based brand, and those with 100 percent pure whey protein isolate such as Isopure and Dymatize. But if you have a favorite that contains 20 to 25 grams of high-quality protein, less than 5 grams of carbs, and less than 2 grams of fats, it's fine to go with that. For ready-to-drink shakes you can grab on the go, some good plant-based ones include Orgain, Vega, and Evolve; for whey-based shakes, consider Muscle Milk, Lean Body, Myoplex, or Syntha-6.

For protein bars, I recommend No Cow, Good2Go (G2G), and thinkThin, followed by One Bar and Quest Bar, and then KIND Protein Bars. All of these bars are best used as snacks before or after a workout—and it's ideal if you can find bars that have 18 grams or more of protein (the KIND Protein Bars are a bit lower than the others with 12 grams of protein but also lower in carbs with 17 grams per bar).

· · ·

EXERCISE BASICS

Regardless of our inherent body types, we all have muscles that are composed of two different types of fibers: Slow-twitch fibers have small motor neurons, produce low tension on the muscle, and are fatigue-resistant (they're great for endurance activities). By contrast, fast-twitch muscles are responsible for strength and power: the type 2A fibers have medium-sized motor neurons, produce high tension, and are somewhat resistant to fatigue (they're responsible for strength output); type 2B fibers, which have large motor neurons and produce very high tension, generate power but fatigue quickly. Our body types can predispose us to have certain muscle fibers that are more dominant than others, so the ratios of these different fiber types can vary from one person to another. Fortunately, the right workouts and training protocol can enhance particular muscle fibers, as you'll see.

When it comes to movement, every little bit counts and the goal is to add more to your life. You'll find specific body-type workout regimens in the chapters that follow, but there are a few principles that are common to all.

+ For cardiovascular exercise—walking, jogging, cycling, swimming, stair-climbing, skating, using cardio machines, or playing movement-related sports (such as soccer or basketball)—intensity is a key concept. When I refer to moderate intensity (such as brisk walking), I mean an intensity that increases your heart rate to 55 to 70 percent of your maximum heart rate (MHR). To figure out what that is, use this formula: subtract your age from 220 to get your MHR, then multiply your MHR by .55 (55 percent) to get the lower end of this range and multiply your MHR by .70 (70 percent) to get the upper end. That's where you want your heart rate while you're exercising at a moderate intensity. Granted, using this approach requires checking your heart rate regularly, which can be a hassle. If you want to keep it simple, you can use the talk test:

you should be able to talk while walking briskly (or cycling or whatever, at a moderate intensity)—but you shouldn't be able to sing. If you can belt out a tune, you need to step up your pace, resistance, or another parameter of intensity.

✧ When it comes to weight training, it's important to choose a weight that allows you to do the desired number of repetitions (reps) with some difficulty but would allow you to do a few more reps on the first set if I really pushed you. Over time, your goal is to add weight and increase resistance, but proper form is essential at every phase. Be patient because building volume and progression is a process that takes time. Many of the programs include compound movements (exercises that use multiple joints and muscles, such as deadlifts and squats with dumbbells) with a focus on building strength and coordination throughout the entire frame, with additional isolation movements (such as biceps curls) to create definition, shape, and symmetry. With each program, you'll want to rest for 60 to 90 seconds between sets, and you'll want to have one rest day between each of your lifting days to allow your muscles sufficient time to recover.

With both cardio workouts and strength training, the overload, adaptation, and progression principles of exercise come into play. When your body is challenged with a given exercise workload (such as lifting a certain amount of weight or jogging at a particular pace), it eventually adapts to the challenge (usually after 8 to 12 weeks). That's a great thing because it means you've made progress and gotten stronger or faster or gained greater endurance, but it also means you're not reaping as many benefits as you previously did from the challenge. At that point, you'll need to create a progression of the load (either the amount of weight or the number of reps, or the pace or intensity of your cardio workout) so you can continue to make progress; otherwise, your fitness benefits can stall and you can grow bored or frustrated. When it's time to increase the challenge, the rule of thumb is to do it by a maximum of 10 to 20 percent per week, whether that means increasing your pace or the duration of your run by that much or adding that much weight or number of reps to your strength-training routine.

The workouts in this book are designed as if you were my client in the gym. They use weights. They use machines. And they rely on body weight. My hope is that you will use this approach at a gym where you'll have more equipment at your disposal and can get the best results. Don't be intimidated; I'll guide you through the workouts and spell out the details so they're crystal clear. You can progress faster and add resistance much more easily when you have access to the equipment of a full gym. So find a club, gym, or other work-out venue where you feel safe and comfortable, and go to it! After a few weeks, the workouts will feel natural and you'll feel in your element; your comfort zone will have broadened. But doing something is always better than noth-ing—so in a pinch you can modify the workouts to your needs and the equip-ment you have available at home and do them there.

· · · · · · · · · A PROPENSITY FOR INTENSITY · · · · · · · · ·

HIGH-INTENSITY INTERVAL TRAINING (HIIT) is a hot concept in the fitness world—and for good reason: you can get a greater bang for your buck with these workouts, especially since they often last just 15 minutes. By alternating short bouts of vigorous exercise with brief periods of active recovery (as in exercising at a slower pace), anaerobic HIIT allows you to torch more calories and push your heart rate more than you could with aerobic steady-state exercise, thus boosting your overall aerobic capacity faster.

As an added perk, you'll crank up the after-burn effect (a.k.a. excess post-exercise oxygen consumption) even more; these terms refer to an increase in the rate at which you burn calories after the workout to help your body recover, cool down, and deal with the hormonal changes the workout produced. Simply put, there's an exponential relationship between exercise intensity and the magnitude of the after-burn effect. So, while any form of aerobic exercise will raise your metabolic rate during the workout and afterwards for a while, HIIT increases these benefits even more. HIIT also confers specific health benefits, including better blood sugar regulation and blood vessel (a.k.a. endothelial) function.

Here's an example of how I introduce HIIT cardio to my clients' programs: after weight training, HIIT cardio is done either on a treadmill or, when the option is available, outside on a level grass surface. This workout can be used for every body type program.

- Do a 30-second sprint at 60 percent of your maximum effort
- Walk for 1 minute at a regular pace
- Do a 30-second sprint at 70 percent of your maximum effort
- Walk for 1 minute at a regular pace
- Do a 30-second sprint at 80 percent (or more) of your maximum effort
- Walk for 1 minute at a regular pace
- Do a 30-second sprint at 80 percent (or more) of your maximum effort
- Walk for 1 minute at a regular pace
- Do a 30-second sprint at 80 percent (or more) of your maximum effort
- Walk for 1 minute at a regular pace

Repeat the intense rotations (80 percent or more of your maximum effort) followed by bouts of active recovery for a total of 12 minutes (15 for advanced exercisers), then finish with a 5-minute cool-down in which you walk at a comfortable pace. After two to four weeks, you can increase the challenge (the progression) by lowering the recovery interval to 30 seconds and/or by increasing the intensity to 90 percent (or more) of your maximum effort for each intense interval. The total time for HIIT cardio doesn't need to exceed 15 minutes, and doing it three or four times a week is plenty. (Advanced HIIT enthusiasts and athletes can train with 45-second sprint intervals at 100 percent maximum effort, with as little as 20-second recovery intervals.)

• • •

When it comes to the diet versus training ratio for achieving optimal results, you'll hear a variety of proportions being thrown around. Some say that losing weight or shedding body fat is 50 percent dependent on diet; others say it's 80. The reality is there's no magical formula. Some people will need to train harder in order to see the results they want, while others will need to alter their diets more dramatically to obtain the results they're pursuing.

The important thing to remember is that each of us spends a limited amount of time each week working out—and a huge amount of time doing other things (including eating). You can't out-train a bad diet so don't even try to. Avoid letting your diet derail your excellent work in the gym or weight room; instead, set your diet up to support your efforts to build muscle and shed body fat.

SUPPORTING PLAYERS

Building a stronger, fitter body, of any type, requires consistent energy and effort, so you'll need to replenish your reserves on the regular. In particular, this means making it a priority to get enough rest and sleep (most people need 7 to 9 hours of good-quality shut-eye per night). Most of the repair of the body's systems, including to your muscles, occurs during sleep, and the brain consolidates new information into memory during sleep; plus, if you don't get enough sleep, that can take a toll on your workouts. Research has found that when adults have their sleep limited to just 5½ hours a night (from 8 hours per night), their physical activity levels decrease by 31 percent and the intensity of their exercise sessions drops by 24 percent. Meanwhile, a study in a 2018 issue of the *Journal of Science and Medicine in Sport* concluded that insufficient sleep impairs maximal muscle strength in compound movements during resistance training.

So forget the adage "You snooze, you lose." If you want to change your body, sleep is your best ally. For one thing, growth hormone, which helps your metabolism function efficiently, is secreted when you sleep; if you don't get enough shut-eye, your resting metabolic rate can suffer. Getting adequate sleep is also important for keeping the hormones that regulate appetite in the proper balance, whereas snoozing too little can promote sneaky, harmful inflammation in your body.

Meanwhile, make an effort to prevent stress from getting the upper hand on you or your life. When you're faced with stress, the sympathetic nervous system activates the body's fight-or-flight response (including the release of cortisol and adrenaline), increasing your heart rate and muscle contractions to prime you to run or fight for your life. This is a valuable response if you're being mugged but not if you're struggling with marital difficulties, money problems, excessive work pressure, or other forms of psychological stress. The thing is, the same physiological stress response hits your brain and body whether you're running from a saber-tooth tiger or feeling panicked about your financial situation. Under the conditions involving psychological stress, cortisol, insulin, and blood sugar (glucose) levels remain high, partly because there's no vigorous physical exertion to burn off the excess cortisol, insulin, and blood glucose. Making matters worse, the continuous release of the stress hormone cortisol can promote the accumulation of body fat. So take regular breaks to decompress—with deep breathing, mindfulness meditation, or whatever works for you—throughout the day. For extra incentive, consider this: a study in a 2017 issue of the *Annals of Behavioral Medicine* found that the mere anticipation of stress makes some people less likely to exercise that day or the next day, which is especially unfortunate since moderate to vigorous exercise can actually relieve stress and boost your ability to cope with whatever comes your way.

Treat yourself as if you were your very own coach, cheerleader, and relaxation therapist: make a conscious effort to restore and recharge your body and mind on a regular basis by handling these lifestyle factors the right way. It's a matter of balance, really: if you're going to push yourself to work out hard and fine-tune your diet in order to transform your body, you'll need to show it some love with ample R & R. That way, you'll be able to build your best body yet while continuously rejuvenating your energy and enthusiasm.

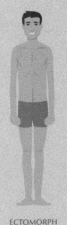

4

ECTOMORPH

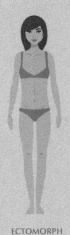

ECTOMORPH

THE ECTOMORPH RX

WHAT DO SUPERMODEL GISELE, FORMER PRESIDENT BARACK Obama, tennis great Roger Federer, Olympic-gold-medal-winning swimmer Michael Phelps, and actors Brad Pitt and Cameron Diaz have in common (besides being famous, of course)? They're all ectomorphs. At any height, ectomorphs tend to appear long and lean with small bones and a relatively low percentage of fat and muscle. They're the ones with the lithe bodies that countless women envy (think: Keira Knightley, Gwyneth Paltrow); on the male side of the ledger, actors Ethan Hawke and Andrew Garfield and singer/songwriter Adam Levine also have the slim builds that are characteristic of ectomorphs. Lanky ectomorphs don't gain weight easily—thanks to their relatively speedy metabolisms—but when they do, it's not usually noticeable with the first 10 pounds. Besides having particularly high thyroid function, these folks often have a higher production of or sensitivity to the stress hormones epinephrine and norepinephrine. Surges of these hormones can lead to peaks and valleys in energy, restlessness, and feelings of lethargy. These stress-hormone fluctuations can compromise endurance, making it difficult for ectomorphs to excel in the weight room or even get through the day in top form.

When their energy is high, ectomorphs are often prone to nonexercise activity thermogenesis (NEAT, for short), a fancy term for burning extra calories through fidgeting and other forms of movement, conscious or not, when they're not actively trying to exercise. You know the type: the woman who's constantly jiggling her foot during a meeting or the guy who has a habit of drumming his fingertips on the desk—people who have trouble sitting still. These are the movers and shakers of the world, the folks who have physical energy to spare so it comes out in (often unintentional) body movements. NEAT is a real thing, so real that research from the Mayo Clinic found that when people engage in fidgeting-like activities while they're seated or standing, they burn up to 50 percent more calories or 80 percent more calories, respectively, during that time period. (Btw, you don't need a fidget-spinner to reap these perks! Just move part of your body.) A review of the effects of NEAT concluded that NEAT movements could add up to expending an extra 2,000 calories per day, beyond your basal metabolic rate (the number of calories your body burns at rest to fulfill basic functions like breathing and keeping your heart beating), depending on your body weight, level of physical activity, and other factors. Given these effects, it's not surprising that research suggests NEAT can make people resistant to gaining body fat even when they overeat. And if you spend more time on your feet than sitting down, you'll naturally burn more calories in a day.

Ectomorphs are sometimes called "hard-gainers" because they can seem to eat whatever they want and/or whenever they want without adding weight to their long, thin physiques. But that doesn't mean they're naturally fit, strong, and/or healthy. Plus, time has a way of catching up to many people, and as ectomorphs get older, they can become "skinny fat," evolving into an ecto-endomorph hybrid thanks to poor eating habits and lack of exercise. Ectomorphs have slender bone structure and small joints, so weight gain tends to be more localized than generalized—fat buildup most commonly occurs in the abdomen and lower back, as well as the chest (especially for men) and upper arms (for women). Unfortunately, these changes can, in turn, increase the risk of developing heart disease, cancer, and other serious health problems, so this isn't just a cosmetic problem. The point is that naturally slender ectomorphs don't get a hall pass that doesn't expire when it comes to diet or physical activity. The quality of these habits still counts!

While people with this body type burn calories easily and rapidly, they typically struggle to gain muscle mass. But it's certainly not impossible for them to do so with the right training regimen and some key dietary changes.

GIVING YOUR BODY WHAT IT NEEDS

On the dietary front, ectomorphs generally rock and roll with more carbohydrates (even a vegan diet), along with a moderate protein and a lower fat intake—a macronutrient distribution of approximately 45 to 55 percent carbs, 25 to 35 percent protein, and 20 percent fat (note: the carb-to-protein ratio can vary, depending on whether the person is trying to slim down or add muscle, but the fat intake should stay low). Since they're naturally thin, ectomorphs are generally inclined to be insulin-sensitive, meaning their bodies are efficient at regulating blood sugar and insulin levels. If you're an ectomorph, this means that your pancreas, which produces insulin, is working well, your other organs are operating efficiently, and consuming carbs doesn't stress out your body. Ectomorphs also typically have a healthy ratio of ghrelin (the so-called "hunger hormone" that stimulates appetite) to leptin (the hormone that signals fullness or satiety); this optimal ratio helps you moderate your calorie intake in ways that allow your body to maintain homeostasis (a consistent internal environment, including hormonal stability). In other words, your total daily calorie consumption is in line with your body's needs.

Consider yourself fortunate in all these respects! This means you probably don't have to be as conscientious (at least right now) with your diet or workout habits as other body types do. If you love pasta, bread, or rice, you can likely have your fill, because your body can probably use these carbs consistently for optimal performance. But even for you, lucky ectomorphs, the quality of your carbohydrates still matters for the sake of your health and energy. So don't give yourself permission to subsist on donuts or cookies; whenever possible, choose performance-enhancing carbs like whole-wheat bread, bean pasta, or brown rice.

Unlike other body types, ectomorphs require less cardiovascular exercise to stay slim. For them, the key to building muscle is to crank up the frequency and intensity of strength-training workouts—by focusing on lifting heavy weights (particularly free weights) three times per week and doing high-intensity interval training (HIIT) two to three times a week (see "A Propensity for Intensity," page 34). An added benefit: lifting weights can stimulate a further increase in insulin sensitivity, allowing you to continue to burn carbs at an enviable rate.

As an example, consider actress Sarah Shahi (who's best known for her roles in the TV shows *Reverie, Person of Interest, Fairly Legal,* and *Life*), who began working with me after having twins. Her goals were to slim down, shape up, and gain muscle strength and definition. Because Sarah has a naturally lean ectomorph body type, she could handle a bit more carbs, so I designed a plan that was 50 percent carbs, 25 percent protein, 25 percent fat (note: we made her fat intake 5 percent higher to fulfill her body's post-baby dietary needs), and 1,800 calories per day. She maximized her nutrition plan five days a week and let herself cut loose and have fun two days a week—so she could enjoy cocktails and ice cream on weekends. Sarah brought the same self-discipline and motivation to her workouts: she did weight-training three times a week for an hour, plus cardio workouts (like kickboxing, walk-to-sprint intervals on the treadmill, or other HIIT) two to three times a week. Within 10 weeks, she lost 12 pounds and gained strength, as well as a tighter, more toned look to her already fit bod.

SLIMMING DOWN, SHAPING UP

For ectomorphs who want to trim body fat and allow their lean muscle to show through more naturally, I recommend sticking with a diet plan that consists of between 1,450 calories (for women and people who are less active) and 1,950 calories (for men, people who are very physically active or already somewhat muscular). For someone who weighs 140 to 200 pounds and expends a moderate amount of energy through physical activity, I'd advise them to consume 100 to 150 grams (400 to 600 calories) of protein per day, 120 to 160 grams (480 to 640 calories) of carbohydrates per day, and 60 to 80 grams (540 to 720 calories) of fat per day. Don't be surprised if you find yourself eating more than you usually do (that happens to many of my clients); the difference here is that you'll be consuming the right combo of calories from wholesome foods at the right times for your body's needs. So you may end up eating more food more often, but your total calorie intake will be the same or lower than what you're used to.

Let's cut to the chase. Here's what a week's worth of meals looks like with this approach:

SUNDAY

Breakfast: 1 to 2 slices Ezekiel bread (toasted), spread with ¼ avocado (mashed), 2 eggs scrambled in 1 tablespoon coconut oil

Snack: Protein shake, ½ banana

Lunch: Greek salad made with 2 cups dark leafy greens, 3 chopped olives, ¼ chopped tomato, ¼ cup chopped cucumber, ¼ cup red pepper chunks, and 1–2 tablespoons apple cider vinegar or lemon juice, topped with 4 ounces grilled chicken

Snack: 1 cup raw green beans with 2 tablespoons hummus

Dinner: 4 ounces grilled or broiled salmon, 1 cup steamed broccoli, 1 small cooked sweet potato

MONDAY

Breakfast: 1 cup cooked oatmeal, 2 tablespoons chopped walnuts, ½ banana (sliced), 1 teaspoon cinnamon

Snack: 2 celery stalks spread with 1 tablespoon almond butter

Lunch: 4 ounces roasted turkey, ½ cup cooked brown rice, 1 cup roasted Brussels sprouts

Snack: Protein shake with ½ cup blueberries

Dinner: Kabobs made with 6 shrimp, chunks of zucchini, mushrooms, and onions, served on ½ cup cooked quinoa

TUESDAY

Breakfast: 2 poached eggs with 1 cup spinach (sautéed in 1 tablespoon coconut oil), 1–2 slices Ezekiel bread (toasted)

Snack: 1 protein bar, ½ cup mango chunks

Lunch: 1 cup lentil salad,* ½ cup cucumber slices

Snack: 1 cup blackberries plus 12 almonds

Dinner: 4 ounces broiled chicken breast, 10 spears steamed asparagus, 1 small cooked sweet potato

WEDNESDAY

Breakfast: 1 cup chia pudding,* mixed with 1 tablespoon chopped nuts and ½ scoop protein powder

Snack: Protein shake with ½ cup raspberries

Lunch: 1 cup butternut squash soup, 1 quinoa–black bean burger with salsa, small salad (mixed greens, sliced tomato, ½ tablespoon avocado oil, 1 tablespoon apple cider vinegar)

Snack: 1 brown-rice cake topped with 1 tablespoon nut butter, ½ banana (sliced)

Dinner: 4 ounces grilled shrimp or scallops stir-fried with 2 cups mixed veggies (broccoli florets, onions, zucchini, spinach, snow peas) in 1 tablespoon sesame oil, served on ½ cup cooked quinoa

THURSDAY

Breakfast: Protein pancakes,* topped with 1 tablespoon almond butter, apple slices

Snack: 1 cup plain Greek or Icelandic yogurt, ½ cup strawberry slices

Lunch: Mix ½ cup tuna with 1 chopped egg and 2 tablespoons of a plain Greek yogurt–mustard mix, wrap in 2 Romaine lettuce leaves

Snack: 2 tablespoons pumpkin seeds, 1 orange

Dinner: 4 ounces broiled grass-fed flank steak, 1 cup cauliflower mash, 1 cup zucchini rounds sautéed in grapeseed oil

FRIDAY

Breakfast: 1 omelet muffin,* 1 slice Ezekiel toast, 1 cup berries

Snack: Protein shake, ½ banana

Lunch: 1 cup black bean or squash soup, ½ turkey sandwich (4 ounces turkey, 3 avocado slices, 1 slice tomato, 1 teaspoon mustard on 1 slice Ezekiel bread)

Snack: 1 cup sugar snap peas with 2 tablespoons hummus

Dinner: 4 ounces grilled salmon, 1 cup roasted cauliflower, ½ cup cooked quinoa

SATURDAY

Breakfast: Butternut squash pancakes,* topped with ¼ cup Icelandic coconut yogurt, 1 tablespoon slivered almonds

Snack: 1 protein bar, ½ cup blueberries

Lunch: 2 cups baby spinach with 4 ounces sautéed organic tofu or tempeh, ½ cup red pepper strips, ½ cup broccoli florets, 1 tablespoon walnut oil; ½ cup cooked brown rice

Snack: 1 hardboiled egg, 1 tablespoon hummus

Dinner: 1 cup turkey chili,* ½ cup cauliflower rice, small salad (mixed greens, sliced tomato, 1 tablespoon balsamic vinaigrette)

Recipes included in Appendix B.

Consistency is important with your eating habits, but you don't want your meals to get monotonous, nor do you want to force yourself to eat foods you don't like. But if you do have meals you're especially crazy about and you are happy to eat frequently, I highly recommend preparing a week's worth at a time (then refrigerating or freezing them), so they're ready to eat when you want them. This way, you can eliminate the stress of cooking or eating out too often. You can also switch out a serving of any of the foods in the meals and replace it with a food from the table below in the same category. But make sure you stick with the recommended serving size—don't just eyeball it because it's easy to underestimate how much food you're taking or eating. Remember, too, that you should consume high protein and high carb meals before and after your workouts, then enjoy moderate protein, moderate carbs, and low fat the rest of the day.

CARBS	PROTEINS	FATS
sweet potatoes	chicken/turkey	nuts
Ezekiel bread	eggs/egg whites	seeds (pumpkin, chia, sprouted)
oats	fish	eggs
brown rice	broccoli/lentils/black beans	coconut oil (hot or cold)
quinoa	protein powder	olive oil (cold)

If you're an ectomorph who wants to lose stubborn body fat, it's wise to build extra muscle mass with a *specific resistance training routine* that provides a mix of both compound movements with heavy weights and a high volume (a.k.a. more reps) of isolation exercises (moves that isolate and directly target the biceps and triceps, for example), done in the right order. Ectomorphs generally have to build up strength, power, and muscle fibers simultaneously, which is no easy feat! The goal for an ecto is to maximize muscular hypertrophy—increasing the number of muscle cells and muscle fiber size. After all, having additional muscle mass actually requires more energy to sustain (which means your metabolic rate will increase), and it will help you stay leaner with an easy-to-maintain regimen for the long haul. By adopting an intense weight-lifting program along with a wholesome diet, ectomorphs will soon notice they can trim unwanted body fat and positively reshape their bodies. Building muscle mass is the key to long-term fat loss. With more muscle, you'll look and feel fitter and better because muscle is denser than body fat is, and it gives your body definition.

IF YOUR WEIGHT is changing by more than two pounds per week in either direction after the first week or two, check your portions to make sure that you're not eating more or less than you think you are. (Get out the food scale and measuring cups and spoons, if need be.) If you're sure your portions are accurate and you're gaining too much weight, try cutting 10 to 20 percent from your food intake across the board. If you're losing more than two pounds per week, try adding 10 to 20 percent to your daily intake. It's important to keep the rate of your weight changes in the healthy zone.

· · ·

THE ECTOMORPH SLIM DOWN, SHAPE UP WORKOUT

For ectomorphs who want to shed some pounds while toning up, the focus is on gaining muscle and doing less cardio. My favorite approach with these folks is to have them do strength training through body-weight exercises while still getting the cardio burn with calisthenic-type moves. You can do this by performing a circuit of 10 full-depth squats, 10 burpees (without push-ups), 10 push-ups, and 10 V-ups in a row, then rest for 30 seconds and repeat. Do five rounds of this (for up to 15 minutes total), two or three times per week.

On the resistance training front, the focus for ectomorphs is on compound movements (exercises that use multiple joints and muscles such as deadlifts and squats with dumbbells), which will promote strength and functionality. On this program, you'll do weight training three times per week with the following pattern. (First, warm up your muscles with a 5-minute stint on a cardio machine, jumping rope, or doing jumping jacks.)

Using the program that follows, choose a weight that feels challenging when you do the desired number of repetitions (reps) but that you could also extend to a few more reps on the first set if I really pushed you. For example, if you can do squats with 10-pound dumbbells for 12 reps but you know you have a few more in you (let's say you would guess 15), then that's a good weight for you to start with. On the other hand, if you can do 10 and maybe force yourself to eke out 12 for the first set, you would not be able to get through all five sets. Remember, the volume (the number of reps times the number of sets you do of an exercise) and your form are more important than the weight you use. You'll find descriptions of all the exercises in Appendix A.

LEGS/SHOULDERS DAY:

5 sets of Weighted Squats (8–12 reps)
3 sets of 20 Leg Presses (on a weight machine)
3 sets of 15 Hamstring Curls (on a weight machine)
3 sets of 20 Walking Lunges with Dumbbells
3 sets of 12 Shoulder Presses with Dumbbells
3 sets of 20 Lateral Raises
3 sets of 10 Front Dumbbell Raises

CHEST/BACK DAY:

3 sets of 8–12 reps Flat Bench Presses
3 sets of 15 Incline Dumbbell Presses
3 sets of 15 Incline Dumbbell Flies
3 sets of Push-Ups to the point of failure
4 sets of 8 Deadlifts
3 sets of 10 Lat Pulldowns (with narrow grip)
3 sets of 12 Bent Rows (with wide grip)
3 sets of 20 Bent-Over Reverse Flies

ARMS/ABS DAY:

3 sets of 10 Biceps Barbell Curls

3 sets of 10 Hammer Curls

3 sets of 15 Preacher Curls

3 sets of 10 Triceps Pushdowns

3 sets of 10 Skull Crushers

3 sets of 15 Overhead Triceps Rope Extensions (or kickbacks)

2 sets of Triceps Dips (as many as you can do at a time)

3 sets of Planks (as long as you can hold them each time)

3 sets of Side Planks (as long as you can hold them on each side)

3 sets of 10 V-Ups, followed immediately by 20 Supermans

With each exercise on each day, rest 60 seconds between each set and include a rest day between each of your lifting days. It's fine to double up your workouts—doing cardio and a strength-training workout on the same day—but not two days in a row.

THE CREATING AND SHAPING MUSCLE PLAN

The key to changing an ectomorph physique is to focus on gaining muscle mass, which requires eating more calories than the body is burning (to gain weight) and doing a strength-training program (to gain muscle, not body fat). What we're doing is essentially forcing a nonmuscular body to grow new muscle cells, which will increase your metabolic rate. Think of this as an investment: the number on the scale may increase by a few pounds—since you'll be adding muscle—but the composition and shape of your body will be much leaner and the strength of your body will be considerably greater.

For ectomorphs who want to gain significant muscle strength and definition, the approach I use with my male clients involves consuming about 2 grams of carbohydrates per pound of total body weight and about 1.5 grams of protein per pound of body weight. This means that a man who's an ectomorph and weighs 150 pounds would consume 300 grams of carbs and 225 grams of protein. Women can apply the same principles to the nutrient breakdown at roughly 75 percent of the man's numbers—225 grams of carbs and 169 grams of protein, for a tall, lean woman who weighs 150 pounds. Depending on a woman's goals, this ratio can be tweaked so that she consumes 1.5–2 grams of carbs per pound of weight and .75 to 1.25 grams of protein per body weight; carbs are especially important for building endurance, and protein is more crucial for building strength and muscle. (Once you have achieved your desired body look and feel, your protein intake can be reduced.)

You can use the weight-loss meal plan as a guide—but you'll want to change your carb servings (rice, quinoa, etc.) to 1 cup instead of ½ cup and your protein servings (fish, poultry, meat, tofu) from 4 ounces to 6 ounces at each meal; your fat intake should remain the same. The goal is to consume 500 more calories per day, from carbs and protein, than on the other plan.

Meanwhile, heavy resistance training is recommended for ectomorphs who want to add strong, sculpted muscle. This involves doing weight training with heavy resistance, mostly keeping reps in the 8 to 12 range, but with occasional 5-rep sets and 20-rep sets (to the point of burnout) to maximize the amount of muscle fibers that are activated. But you need to be careful about not overdoing it with cardio workouts and you may need to avoid cardio entirely during this "muscle-growing" phase; otherwise, it will be difficult to add muscle mass because you'll be burning calories for energy instead of putting them toward muscle growth.

For men or women who are "skinny" or "lanky" and want to add muscle mass, I recommend increasing your daily protein intake and consuming a large portion of carbs (say, 50 grams) and protein (say, 30 grams) with the meal before training and again after your resistance-training workouts. The reasons: consuming carbs before a workout helps fuel optimal energy levels by providing instant energy as well as sending extra energy to be stored as glycogen; consuming carbs after a workout helps replenish your glycogen stores, as well as raising your insulin level, thereby shuttling nutrients to your muscles to begin the repair processes. Similarly, consuming protein before and after your workouts provides your muscles with the amino acids they need to function and create new muscle cells and fibers. To avoid the hassle factor of having to prepare meals five or six times per day (I'm assuming you don't have a personal chef), protein shakes or smoothies are easy, convenient ways to add extra protein to your diet. Remember, this is a good way to supplement your protein intake; protein shakes shouldn't become a staple of your diet (that's what real food is for).

When I started working with Jack Barakat, lead guitarist and backing vocalist for pop-rock band All Time Low, in 2017, he wanted to add chiseled muscle to his long and lanky ectomorph frame (he's 6'3"). I encouraged him to be conscious about keeping his fat intake low and to keep his intake of good-quality carbs and proteins high (for a breakdown of 40 percent carbs, 40 percent protein, 20 percent fat). Once I got him lifting weights three times a week, focusing on heavy compound lifts (such as deadlifts and bench presses), and doing HIIT body-weight workouts twice a week for 15 minutes at a time, within months he gained serious strength. On day one, he could do 3 push-ups and bench press 65 pounds; now, he can do 50 push-ups and bench press 165 pounds. Meanwhile, his Instagram account lit up with fans commenting on his "guitar jacked arms" as he played to crowds of 20,000 during the band's Warped Tour. It's an impressive transformation, any way you slice it!

For ectomorphs who don't want or need to slim down but do want to add muscle mass, strength, and definition to their frames, a smartly executed strength-training program is key! In particular, focusing on the volume and frequency of resistance training is especially important to build new muscle tissue. The latter isn't easy for ectomorphs, who generally start weightlifting programs feeling rather weak and having little muscular endurance. To change that, the frequency and consistency of your strength-building workouts are crucial. With a muscle-building exercise program designed for ectomorphs, the goal is to maximize the body's anabolic state, in which your body is growing, repairing, and strengthening muscle tissue. An added perk: resistance training also increases your bone density and the strength of your connective tissue.

When you start the program that follows, choose a weight that feels challenging when you do the desired number of repetitions (reps) but that you could also extend to a few more reps on the first set if you were pushed to. For example, if you can do Flat Bench Presses with 85 pounds for 12 reps but you know you have a few more in you (let's say 15), then that's a good weight for you to start with. On the other hand, if you can do 10 and maybe force yourself to eke out 12 for the first set, you would *not* be able to get through all 3 sets. Remember: the volume (the number of reps times the number of sets you do of an exercise) and your form are more important than the weight you use.

LEGS/ABS DAY:

5 sets of 12 Weighted Squats
3 sets of 12 Romanian Deadlifts
3 sets of 20 Squat Jumps
3 sets of 12 Walking Lunges with dumbbells
3 sets of 10 Leg Presses (on a weight machine)

3 sets of Planks (holding each one as long as you can)
3 sets of Side Planks (holding each one as long as you can on each side)
3 sets of 15 V-Ups, immediately followed by 20 Supermans

CHEST/BACK DAY:

5 sets of 8–12 Incline Bench Presses

3 sets of 10 Flat Bench Presses with dumbbells

3 sets of 12 Dumbbell Pec Flies

3 sets of 12 Dips (use machine that assists)

3 sets of Push-Ups to the point of failure

5 sets of 5–12 Lat Pulldowns (start with light weight and high reps, add weight each set)

4 sets of 6–10 Bent Rows

4 sets of 8 Deadlifts

3 sets of 6–8 One-Arm Dumbbell Rows

SHOULDERS/ARMS DAY:

3 sets of 6–10 Shoulder Presses with Dumbbells

3 sets of 20 Lateral Raises

3 sets of 10 Front Dumbbell Raises

3 sets of 15 seated Military Presses on a Smith machine

With the exercises that follow, you'll want to do 10–15 reps per set, with 3-second negatives. This means slowing down the lowering or downward part of the lift—the eccentric phase, which is what causes the muscles to adapt and get stronger—to 3 seconds.

3 sets of alternating Standing Barbell Curls and Skull Crushers

3 sets of alternating Dumbbell Biceps Curls and Triceps Rope Pushdowns

3 sets of alternating Hammer Curls and Triceps Dips

With each exercise on each day, rest 60 seconds between each set and include a rest day between each of your lifting days. It's fine to double up your workouts—doing cardio and a strength-training workout on the same day—but not two days in a row.

BODY-WEIGHT HIIT WORKOUT:

Twice a week, perform the following HIIT segment, using your body weight. This will be your only cardio routine. This HIIT-style workout is very efficient at burning a lot of calories in just a short time. Perform all the reps of each exercise without stopping, then immediately move on to the next exercise.

20 Squats

10 Push-Ups

30-second Plank, 30-second Side Plank on each side (for 1½ minutes total)

30-second Mountain Climbers

20 Supermans

10 Burpees (without Push-Ups)

Take a 30-second break then repeat this sequence as many times as you can in 15 minutes.

THE PAYOFFS

Look, I realize all of this may sound a bit overwhelming, especially if you're relatively new to working out regularly. But you'll get the hang of it quickly and you have so much to gain with this plan. In the short term, you'll get an immediate rush from the boost in circulation and the release of endorphins that's very gratifying and makes you feel happier and less stressed. Within two weeks, you'll notice considerable progress and gains in muscle strength if you do these workouts consistently. And you'll see the difference on your frame: tightness and firmness will appear in new places and you'll start to notice muscle definition you didn't have before. As you begin to feel and look stronger and fitter, you'll gain confidence in your body and mind, which will put some extra pep in your step.

5

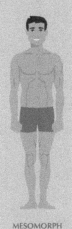

MESOMORPH

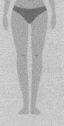

MESOMORPH

THE MESOMORPH RX

LIKE IT OR NOT, MESOMORPHS TEND TO HAVE ATHLETIC BUILDS, with high muscle mass; strong, dense bones; and broad shoulders. They're often larger or broader in the chest but fairly lean all over (that means lower body fat), and they have no trouble gaining muscle mass. This makes perfect sense considering that mesomorphs (like Jennifer Garner, Angela Bassett, Madonna, tennis champ Serena Williams, Mark Wahlberg, Dwayne "The Rock" Johnson, and actor/former California governor Arnold Schwarzenegger) tend to have higher percentages of testosterone and growth hormone, which predisposes them to muscle gain and lower body fat. Their bodies are powerful and strong. In fact, mesomorphs are both loved and hated for their physiques because they have very few "trouble spots": fat is fairly evenly distributed on their bodies, and even then, it appears more as "bulk" or a thin layer of fat on top of developed muscle. These folks typically have relatively thick midsections and legs, so any visible areas of weight gain tend to be on the legs, buttocks, and stomach.

When it comes to food choices, mesomorphs have it relatively easy. They thrive on a well-balanced diet with approximately 40 percent carbohydrates, 30 percent protein, and 30 percent fat (if the goal is to maintain their shape). Since mesomorphs have good insulin sensitivity along with high levels of muscle, this macronutrient ratio fuels their performance, provides energy, and repairs muscle in ways that are exactly in line with their body's needs. Carbs provide glucose for energy production and the replenishment of glycogen (stored glucose) after exercise; protein helps with muscle growth and repair; and healthy fats (like nuts, seeds, olive oil, fatty fish, and avocado) promote satiety and the absorption of fat-soluble vitamins. But mesomorphs have more wiggle room than other body types do and can get away with more frequent indulgences (of carbs or fats, for example) without setting their bodies up for significant (unwanted) consequences. They enjoy efficient leptin-to-ghrelin ratios, which means their hunger is well regulated, as their bodies know what they want and when. Because of their higher percentage of lean muscle mass, mesomorphs tend to need slightly more calories (perhaps 200 to 300 more per day) than endomorphs do; that's because muscle burns more calories than body fat does, so it requires more calories to maintain.

Since their metabolisms are so active, mesomorphs should consume smaller, more frequent meals every few hours—that's the approach my meso clients find to be the most comfortable and successful for them. Whether or not eating more frequently helps improve weight control or body composition hasn't been definitively decided by scientific research (though it looks doubtful). But a strong case has been made for this eating pattern's having positive effects on cholesterol and insulin levels, preserving lean muscle mass when cutting calories, and decreasing hunger and improving appetite control.

Even so, the best way to eat is the one that works for you. If you want to eat frequently to stay satisfied and energized, go with smaller meals more often. If you like bigger portions, that's fine, but have them less frequently. So long as you eat high-quality foods that fulfill your body's macronutrient requirements, you'll be in good shape.

One exception that's worth noting: To maintain a lean physique and maximize muscle while burning fat, mesomorphs do very well with a concept called "carb timing." This involves placing your carbohydrate portions primarily in the meals directly before and after your workouts. With this approach, carbs will fuel your workout and aid in your post-workout recovery by shuttling protein and other key nutrients into your muscles afterwards. Making sure your other meals have a higher focus on protein and fat with a lower carb content will help keep your insulin levels stable, which will lead to more controlled energy as well as less fat storage.

You may have read about an eating style that's been dubbed IIFYM (short for If It Fits Your Macros), which has taken the Internet by storm. The idea is that as long as you eat a set amount of fat, carbs, and protein every day, your meals can basically be a free-for-all after that. If, on a given day, you consume a protein shake, two slices of pizza, a salad with chicken, and two tacos, and this makes your protein, carbs, and fat intake total up to the proper numbers, you've hit your target. With the IIFYM approach, there are no "good" or "bad" choices; any food is fair game, as long as you hit your daily totals for macronutrients. It's like getting a hall pass that doesn't expire. While this approach may seem tailor-made for mesomorphs, I'm not a fan, and here's why: if you want to achieve and maintain good health and a fit body, this approach can come back to bite you in the long run because the quality of your nutrient intake really does matter! If you consume lots of artificial ingredients and fake sugars, starchy carbs with little to no nutritional value (at least compared to veggies), and protein and fat from fried or high-fat foods, this can have lasting effects on your hormones and physical well-being. (That said, I tell clients that IIFYM is the perfect tool to use on vacation, when you want to let loose and enjoy yourself.)

MESOMORPHS IN ACTION

Mesomorphs often have a love/hate relationship with health and fitness. Because they're naturally strong and sturdy, many sports come easily to them but their interest or progress in them can fizzle. Regimented training and eating can be hard to sustain for people who get results quickly. With their strong and powerful frames, mesomorphs' bodies are generally dominant with fast-twitch muscles. The good news is that as a result, they excel at bodybuilding and strength- or power-based sports (such as soccer, rugby, and hockey), because they can recruit muscle fibers to put out force quickly and with great strength for a moderate time period. The bad news: since mesomorphs have fewer slow-twitch muscle fibers (they have a high ratio of fast-twitch muscle fibers to slow-twitch muscle fibers), they have lower endurance levels to begin with, which can lead to frustration or fitness plateaus if they don't manage their training properly.

Indeed, mesomorphs tend to plateau in fitness benefits more quickly than other body types do, for a variety of reasons, so it's wise for these folks to keep changing up their workout styles. (In fact, if you hit a fitness plateau, take that as a cue that this is a good time to focus on developing your slow-twitch muscle fibers and endurance performance, which will ultimately shock your body into getting fitter.) To reach their optimal fitness potential, short, intense workout sessions—like high-intensity interval training (HIIT), sprints, or kickboxing—are ideal for mesomorphs. These bodies naturally excel at powerful, explosive movements, but they can tire quickly. Doing short, intense workouts maximizes the bang you, as a mesomorph, can get for your buck (your effort), because you'll be using the aerobic, anaerobic, and musculoskeletal systems efficiently to create body synergy that results in maximum fat loss and muscle gain.

But cardio and strength-training exercises, especially compound movements (such as push-ups with rows, squats with biceps curls, and lateral lunges with chest presses) are equally important for the sake of your endocrine (hormone), cardiovascular, and respiratory systems. In particular, compound strength-training movements recruit more muscle fibers, challenge your core, require more proprioception (the sense you use to understand the relative position of your body parts), and stimulate the central nervous system more than other exercises do. This stimulates a greater secretion of growth hormone and testosterone, key hormones for creating muscle, burning fat, and slowing the aging process. (Don't panic, ladies: increasing your testosterone levels this way won't give you a deep voice or hair growth in unwanted places.)

Mesomorphs really do well with periodization-based training. With fitness, periodization means breaking down a long-term goal into distinctly different training phases to achieve it, based on the assumption that this approach will yield better results than a constant routine that's repeated over and over again. For mesomorphs it's a good idea to change training phases every two to three months, even if the change just involves reps and/or the exercise order. Within these phases, we'd likely change the volume of total sets and reps, the style of exercise, and even the nutritional approach that supports these workouts. For example, a plan might consist of six weeks of using heavy weights, followed by a one-week break, followed by a four-week endurance and cardio phase then a one-week rest, then a six- to eight-week phase of bodybuilding training for aesthetic purposes and high-intensity interval cardio workouts. That's just one example. The program can be tweaked based on whether your goals are performance-based or aesthetically based, but the basic idea is that you want to continue changing your training program to continue varying the challenges to your body.

To be efficient at training and create body changes more quickly, mesomorphs also can leverage their fast-twitch muscle fibers and do compound movements (such as squats, deadlifts, and bench presses), explosive plyometric movements (like squat or box jumps, HIIT cardio), and other cardio and resistance training that's focused on power rather than endurance. Additional work with isolation movements (exercises that isolate the specific muscle groups you want to build, both in strength and for aesthetic purposes, like biceps curls and triceps dips) and lengthy cardio sessions (for health perks or pleasure) are welcome additions, but they're not essential.

SLIMMING DOWN, SHAPING UP

Not long ago, I had an online client in Europe who was 34 and almost a pure mesomorph, but with a few endomorphic qualities. He had been working an office job for 10 years and had fallen into some suboptimal habits—as in, no real nutrition plan or workout regimen. He was still strong, but he had little muscle definition and noticeable excess body fat. I had him do something similar to the plan that follows, and he was able to drop from 221 pounds to 192 on his 6' frame; he also lowered his body fat from 27 percent to 15 percent in six months. At that point, he felt and looked like a totally different human. No exaggeration!

For mesomorphs who want to slim down, it helps to tinker with the macronutrient breakdown that's usually optimal for maintaining this body type. By shifting to getting 30 percent of their daily calories from carbs, 35 percent from protein, and 35 percent from fat, mesomorphs can improve their insulin sensitivity, maximize their muscle growth and metabolic rate, and shed body fat fairly easily. For someone who weighs 140 to 200 pounds and expends a moderate amount of energy through physical activity, I'd advise them to consume 100 to 150 grams (400 to 600 calories) of protein per day, 100 to 140 grams (400 to 560 calories) of carbohydrates per day, and 60 to 80 grams (540 to 720 calories) of fat per day. It's ideal if they can consume slightly more carbs at breakfast and before and after their workouts to keep their energy and performance revved. Their total daily calorie intake will be between 1,500 and 2,300, depending on their starting weight, their level of physical activity, and their body composition (those with more muscle need more calories). The great news for mesomorphs is these percentages can be off a bit and they'll still get the results they want because their insulin sensitivity and metabolisms are so high functioning.

Here's what a week's worth of meals looks like with this approach:

SUNDAY

Breakfast: Protein pancakes,* topped with 1 tablespoon almond butter, 1 cup berries

Snack: Protein shake, ½ apple

Lunch: 1 cup gazpacho, cooked 4-ounce turkey burger served on ½ cup cooked quinoa with chopped avocado and tomato

Snack: 1 cup raw sugar snap peas with 2 tablespoons hummus

Dinner: 6 large grilled shrimp, 1 cup cauliflower rice (cooked with ¼ chopped onion, ½ chopped carrot, ½ chopped red pepper, ¾ teaspoon extra-virgin olive oil, seasonings of choice), 10 steamed asparagus spears

MONDAY

Breakfast: 1 cup plain Greek yogurt with ¾ cup raspberries, 10 almonds, 2 tablespoons low-sugar granola

Snack: 1 protein bar, ½ banana

Lunch: Salad with leafy greens, ½ cup edamame, chopped celery, sliced mushrooms, broccoli florets, ¼ avocado (diced), 1 tablespoon balsamic vinaigrette, 4 ounces cooked salmon

Snack: 1 cup blackberries, 12 almonds

Dinner: 4 ounces broiled flank steak; 2 cups zucchini sautéed with shallots; 1 small cooked sweet potato

TUESDAY

Breakfast: 1 cup cooked oatmeal topped with ½ cup blueberries, 1 tablespoon chopped walnuts, ½ tablespoon chia seeds, ¼ teaspoon cinnamon; hardboiled egg

Snack: 1 protein bar, ½ cup melon chunks

Lunch: Salad with lots of leafy greens, cut-up beets, apple slices, ½ cup chickpeas, 1 tablespoon vinaigrette, 4 ounces grilled chicken

Snack: ½ cup roasted chickpeas, 12 almonds

Dinner: 4 ounces roasted rainbow trout, ½ cup cooked quinoa, 2 cups shaved zucchini, summer squash, radish, and carrot, mixed with chopped dill, 1 teaspoon extra-virgin olive oil, ½ teaspoon rice wine vinegar

WEDNESDAY

Breakfast: 2 eggs scrambled with 1 cup chopped spinach, 1 tablespoon coconut oil, 1–2 slices Ezekiel bread (toasted)

Snack: Protein shake with ½ cup strawberry slices

Lunch: 2 cups mixed leafy greens, ½ cup sliced hearts of palm, ½ cup cucumber chunks, 4 ounces grilled or canned salmon, ½ cup cooked quinoa, 1–1½ tablespoons vinaigrette

Snack: 10 almonds, 1 small pear

Dinner: 4 ounces roasted chicken breast, with ½ cup cooked brown rice, ½ cup roasted butternut squash, ½ cup roasted red pepper strips, drizzled with 1 tablespoon grapeseed oil

THURSDAY

Breakfast: 1 cup cooked oatmeal, 2 tablespoons chopped walnuts, ½ cup roasted nectarine or peach slices,* 1 teaspoon cinnamon

Snack: 1 brown-rice cake topped with 1 tablespoon almond butter, ½ banana (sliced)

Lunch: 1 cup lentil soup,* ½ sandwich (½ cup roasted veggies, 2 avocado slices, 1 slice tomato, 1 teaspoon hummus on 1 slice Ezekiel bread)

Snack: 2 tablespoons pumpkin seeds, 1 orange

Dinner: 1 cup turkey chili,* ½ cup broccoli rice, small salad (mixed greens, sliced tomato, 1 tablespoon balsamic vinaigrette)

FRIDAY

Breakfast: Morning parfait,* 1 slice Ezekiel bread (toasted), spread with ⅛ to ¼ avocado (mashed)

Snack: 1 protein bar, ½ cup blueberries

Lunch: 1 3-inch-square piece of veggie frittata,* 1 slice Ezekiel bread (toasted), side salad

Snack: Cucumber slices with 2 tablespoons hummus

Dinner: 4 ounces grilled or roasted Arctic char fillet, 1½ cups roasted veggies (cauliflower, zucchini, peppers), ½ cup cooked quinoa

SATURDAY

Breakfast: Huevos rancheros,* green juice*

Snack: Protein shake, ½ banana

Lunch: 1 cup turkey chili,* ½ cup cauliflower rice, small salad (mixed greens, sliced tomato, 1 tablespoon balsamic vinaigrette)

Snack: 14 walnut halves, ½ cup raspberries

Dinner: 4 ounces broiled halibut or sea bass, 1 cup roasted Brussels sprouts, leafy green salad with sliced tomato and cucumber, drizzled with 1 tablespoon extra-virgin olive oil and 1 tablespoon balsamic vinegar

* Recipes included in Appendix B.

You can switch out a serving of any of the foods in the suggested meals and replace it with a food from the table below in the same category. But make sure you stick with the recommended serving size—don't just eyeball it because it's easy to underestimate how much food you're taking or eating.

CARBS	PROTEINS	FATS
sweet potatoes	chicken/turkey	nuts
Ezekiel bread	eggs/egg whites	seeds (pumpkin, chia, sprouted)
oats	fish	eggs
brown rice	broccoli/lentils/black beans	coconut oil (hot or cold)
quinoa	protein powder	olive oil (cold)

· TROUBLESHOOTING TIPS ·

IF YOUR WEIGHT is changing by more than two pounds per week in either direction after the first week or two, check your portions to make sure that you're not eating more or less than you think you are. (Get out the food scale and measuring cups and spoons, if need be.) If you're sure your portions are accurate and you're gaining too much weight, try cutting 10 to 20 percent from your food intake across the board. If you're losing more than two pounds per week, try adding 10 to 20 percent to your daily intake. It's important to keep the rate of your weight changes in the healthy zone.

• • •

THE MESOMORPH SLIM DOWN, SHAPE UP WORKOUT

Because of their naturally muscular body compositions, many mesomorphs don't *need* to do steady-state cardio workouts to lose body fat. Instead, an intense strength-training routine with weights and high-intensity interval training is more than enough to stimulate muscle growth and efficient fat burning. But cardio workouts do bring another set of benefits to your cardiorespiratory systems and your brain function, so it's fine to engage in brisk walking or hiking for 30 to 45 minutes, three to five times a week, and/or HIIT sprints or calisthenics circuits for 15 minutes, two or three times per week, either on their own or after a strength-training session. As a mesomorph gets leaner, I definitely recommend adding cardio workouts to the program so you can add more calories to your meals and still reach and maintain your fitness goals.

On the resistance-training front, the focus for mesomorphs is on compound movements, which will promote strength and functionality. With the workout that follows, you should expect to feel a little tired and sore afterwards, at least the first few times, but you'll start to feel better and stronger after each session after the first two weeks. This is a workout that will prime your body to shed fat and bring out your inherent muscle definition and strength. If they're new to strength training, some women worry that they'll build big, bulky muscles; that won't happen with this program, unless you start lifting seriously heavy weight and consuming a lot more calories. Stick to the plan and you'll be good.

On this program, you'll do weight training three times per week with the following pattern. (First, warm up your muscles with a 5-minute stint on a cardio machine, doing burpees, or jumping rope.) Choose a weight where doing the desired number of repetitions (reps) feels difficult but not impossible on the first set. You'll find descriptions of all the exercises in Appendix A.

LEGS/ABS DAY:

For each move, follow a tempo of 2 seconds to lift then lower each weight (or vice versa) with no pause in between.

4 sets of 12 reps Weighted Squats

3 sets of 12 Single-Leg Romanian Deadlifts

3 sets of 20 Squat Jumps

4 sets of 15 Walking Lunges with dumbbells

3 sets of 20 Hamstring Curls (on a machine)

3 sets of Planks (as long as you can hold them each time)

3 sets of Side Planks (as long as you can hold them on each side)

3 sets of 10 V-Ups, followed immediately by 20 Supermans

With each exercise on each day, rest 60 to 90 seconds between each set and include a rest day between each of your lifting days. It's fine to double up your workouts—doing cardio and a strength-training workout on the same day—but not two days in a row.

CHEST/BACK DAY:

3 sets of 12 Incline Bench Presses

3 sets of 15 Flat Dumbbell Bench Presses

3 sets of 12 Dumbbell Flies

3 sets of Push-Ups (as many as you can do; it's okay to do them on your knees)

3 sets of 12 reps Lat Pulldowns (or Pull-Ups using a pull-up machine, if you prefer)

3 sets of 10 Bent Rows

3 sets of 10 Traditional Deadlifts

3 sets of 15 Bent-Over Reverse Flies

With each exercise on each day, rest 60 seconds between each set and include a rest day between each of your lifting days. It's fine to double up your workouts—doing cardio and a strength-training workout on the same day—but not two days in a row.

Finish with a 15-minute HIIT workout.

SHOULDERS/ARMS DAY:

4 sets of 15 Shoulder Presses with Dumbbells

3 sets of 20 Lateral Raises

3 sets of 10 Front Dumbbell Raises

3 sets of 10 Standing Biceps Curls

2 sets of 15 Hammer Curls

3 sets of 12 Preacher Curls

3 sets of 12 Overhead Triceps Extensions

2 sets of 15 Triceps Kickbacks

3 sets of 12 Triceps Pushdowns

With each exercise on each day, rest 60 seconds between each set and include a rest day between each of your lifting days. It's fine to double up your workouts—doing cardio and a strength-training workout on the same day—but not two days in a row.

Finish with a 15-minute HIIT workout.

THE BUILDING AND SHAPING MUSCLE PLAN

When I started working with actress Danielle Fishel (who's perhaps best known for her roles on *Boy Meets World* and *Girl Meets World*, as well as for hosting *The Dish*), she wanted to trim her waistline to appear less boxy. Though quite petite (she's 5'1"), Danielle, a pure mesomorph, came to me with strong, muscular arms, even though she hadn't been training. On day one, she said, "I could probably be a bodybuilder if I wanted—my body grows muscles. But I am getting married and need to slim up and not look like a she-beast." To help her body tighten up and tone up, we focused on a combination of weight training three times per week with HIIT cardio for

15 minutes at the end of a 40-minute weight session. I also wanted her to do as much low-intensity cardio in the fat-burning zone as she could fit into her daily schedule, with a goal of at least three times a week, to burn an extra 300 calories or so on those days. She found a way to do this five times per week by walking her dog for 30 minutes—a win-win for Danielle and her dog!

Meanwhile, we trimmed her carb intake and increased her intake of protein and healthy fats, getting her as close as possible to the 40 percent carbs, 30 percent protein, and 30 percent fat breakdown with 1,600 to 1,800 calories per day, depending on whether it was a training day. Within four months, she went from being able to do 0 pull-ups to nailing 5 at a time, dropping 10 pounds from her 5'1" figure and toning up. It was an impressive body transformation, to say the least!

Both the fitness model world and Hollywood use two phrases a lot—"bulking" and "cutting," which can sound like scary terms to outsiders. Don't be fazed! "Bulking" really just means adding muscle, while "cutting" refers to losing body fat while maintaining muscle. Both of these goals are easy for mesomorphs to achieve, especially compared to endomorphs, who risk adding weight and fat while "bulking," and ectomorphs, who can damage their bodies with "cutting" and end up looking weak and skinny. As a result, mesomorphs have the easiest time of all body types at achieving a body recomposition (a.k.a. recomp), which means adding muscle and losing fat simultaneously.

For mesomorphs who want to build muscle strength, endurance, and definition, but don't want or need to shed much body fat, a 40-30-30 percentage split from carbs, protein, and fat is the sweet spot so you'll have plenty of fuel to build the muscle mass and definition you want. You can use the weight-loss meal plan as a guide—but you'll want to change your carb servings (rice, quinoa, etc.) to 1 cup instead of ½ cup and your protein servings (fish, poultry, meat) from 4 ounces to 6 ounces at each meal; your fat intake should remain the same. The goal is to consume 300 to 500 more calories per day, from carbs and protein, than on the other plan.

On this muscle-building program, you'll do weight training four times per week with the following pattern. (First, warm up your muscles with a 5-minute stint on a cardio machine, doing burpees, or jumping rope.) Choose a weight where doing the desired number of repetitions (reps) feels difficult but not impossible on the first set. For each move, follow a tempo of 2 seconds to lift then lower each weight (or vice versa) with no pause in between.

LEGS/SHOULDERS DAY:

Do the following moves sequentially, including a 60- to 90-second break between each set.

3 sets of 20 Jump Squats

3 sets of 10 Barbell Squats

2 sets of 20 Walking Lunges with dumbbells

3 sets of 10 Stiff-Legged Deadlifts

3 sets of 10 Thrusters

3 sets of 15 Shoulder Presses with dumbbells

3 sets of 20 Lateral Raises

3 sets of 10 Upright Rows

2 sets of 20 Front Dumbbell Raises

CHEST/TRICEPS DAY:

Do the following moves sequentially, including a 60- to 90-second break between each set.

3 sets of 10 Flat Bench Presses

3 sets of 15 Incline Dumbbell Bench Presses

3 sets of 20 Dumbbell Flies

3 sets of Push-Ups (as many as you can do; it's fine to be on your knees)

3 sets of 20 Triceps Pushdowns

3 sets of 10 Skull Crushers

3 sets of as many Triceps Dips as you can do

End with a 15-minute HIIT workout.

BACK/BICEPS DAY:

Do the following moves sequentially, including a 60- to 90-second break between each set.

4 sets of 10 Traditional Deadlifts

3 sets of 10 Bent Rows

3 sets of 12 Lat Pulldowns (or Pull-Ups or using a pull-up machine if you prefer)

3 sets of 15 Bent-Over Reverse Flies

3 sets of 15 Standing Biceps Curls

3 sets of 10 Hammer Curls

3 sets of 12 Preacher Curls

End with a 15-minute HIIT workout.

FULL-BODY DAY:

With the compound movements that follow, take a 2-minute break after each set, then do another set until you've completed three; then move on to the next exercise and repeat this pattern.

3 sets of 5–8 Flat Bench Presses

3 sets of 5–8 Deadlifts

3 sets of 5–8 Shoulder Presses with Dumbbells

CIRCUIT:

After finishing the heavy lifting, do the following circuit of exercises, with 20-second breaks between each type of exercise.

10 Push-Ups

20 Squats

20 Dumbbell Curls

20 Triceps Dips

End with a 1-minute Plank then move into 30 seconds of Side Planks on
each side. Rest 1 minute; repeat 3 times.

BODY-WEIGHT HIIT WORKOUT:

Twice a week, perform the following HIIT segment, using your own body
weight. This will be your only cardio routine. This is a HIIT-style
workout, and it's very efficient at burning a lot of calories in just a short
time. Perform all the reps of each exercise without stopping, then immediately move on to the next exercise.

20 Squats

10 Push-Ups

30-second Plank, 30-second Side Planks on each side (for 1½ minutes
total)

30 seconds of Mountain Climbers

20 Supermans

10 Burpees (without Push-Ups)

Take a 30-second break then repeat this sequence as many times as you
can in 15 minutes.

Alternatively, you can do **hill sprints** (I personally like exercising outside
a lot more, but you can use a machine if you'd prefer), which are one
of my favorite all-around HIIT workouts, especially for mesomorphs:

Max effort sprint (uphill or on incline) for 20 seconds

Jog back for 15 seconds then walk for 15 seconds

Max effort sprint for 25 seconds

Jog back for 15 seconds then walk for 15 seconds

Max effort sprint (uphill or on incline) for 30 seconds
Jog back for 15 seconds then walk for 15 seconds

Repeat this cycle 3 to 4 times, allowing yourself a little extra break time
(up to 1 minute maximum) as needed. Try to work up to 15 minutes of
these hill sprints while paying the most attention to really going all out
on the sprint part.

THE PAYOFFS

Whether you choose the slim-down or muscle-up plan, you should see boosts
in your muscle strength by the week and increases in your muscle definition
and overall tone by the month. Hit the pause button periodically on your busy
life and take a moment to notice these changes: see them, feel them, and appreciate them—and enjoy the confidence boost that comes with them! *You've earned it!*

But don't just sit back and rest on your ass. Since muscle growth comes
relatively easily to mesomorphs, you can trade cardio workouts or periodization strength-training workouts for your usual ones, now and then, to keep
things fresh and effective in the fitness department. In fact, I encourage you to
do so, not only for the sake of your state of mind and continued motivation but
also so that you don't hit or stay on a fitness plateau. That's something mesomorphs are particularly susceptible to—it's the price you lucky mesomorphs
pay for having bodies that respond and adapt to physical challenges so well
and so quickly. So continue to push yourself and shake things up on the regular so you can keep reaping the get-fit, feel-good perks from your workouts.
You've got the power to do so—wield it wisely!

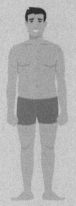

ENDOMORPH

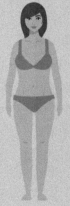

ENDOMORPH

THE ENDOMORPH RX

CURVES ARE SEXY. FULLNESS IS SENSUOUS. MUSCLES ARE POWER-ful and impressive. Even with so many desirable physical traits, endomorphs tend to be pretty hard on themselves (in my experience). This is somewhat understandable given that we live in a culture that's obsessed with thinness, but it's still a shame because endos, as I like to call them, have so many excellent attributes: the potential to be super-strong athletes, with explosive power in sports and excellent balance capabilities, for starters. Performance wise, research has found that endomorphs are capable of dominating a wide range of sports, including water polo, surfing, judo, and discus throwing. From an aesthetic point of view, they have the ability to develop shapely or curvy physiques that are also well defined.

Often described as stout or round, curvaceous or voluptuous, endomorphs tend to have a medium-to-large bone structure, with more of their weight in their lower abdomen, hips, and thighs. They often have a higher percentage of body fat than other types, and they tend to gain weight easily, which is why they may find themselves on the rounder or softer side even if they're not overweight. While endomorphs (like celebrities Jennifer Lopez, Beyoncé, Sofía Vergara, Queen Latifah, Chris Pratt, Russell Crowe, and James Corden) have no trouble gaining muscle, it's often harder for them to lose body fat, partly because they tend to have slower metabolisms. While their bodies are all a bit different, Chris Pratt, Russell Crowe, and James Corden have sturdy physiques, with thick midsections and rounder bodies, characteristics that are typical of male endomorphs.

In fact, research has found that while women who are endomorphs tend to consume fewer calories than their peers who are ectomorphs or mesomorphs, they have a harder time maintaining an ideal body weight, which has to be frustrating. When endomorphs gain weight, prime trouble spots include the abdomen (hello, muffin top!) and butt, but the arms can become flabby and the legs can become jiggly as well. If an endomorph with the same height and weight as his or her friends who are mesomorphs eats the same meals as those friends, the endomorph will hold onto more body fat. This is totally unfair, I know, but it is what it is: simply put, endomorphs have different responses to certain foods than people with other body types do. But if you are an endomorph, don't give up because it is possible for endomorphs to bring out the best in their physiques—with the right dietary approach and plenty of fat-burning aerobic exercise, plus strength training three times a week. Even if the goal isn't to shed body weight, you can achieve a shift in body composition with the right adjustments to your lifestyle.

Before we delve into the details on how to do that, let's take a closer look at what's going on inside endomorphs. Typically, endomorphs have slower sympathetic nervous systems (which means it takes more to mobilize the body's fight-or-flight response) and a greater propensity toward insulin resistance. Endomorphs naturally have a higher percentage of body fat and slower metabolisms, partly due to genetic factors and partly because they're likely to be somewhat insulin-resistant. High insulin levels can bring on intense food cravings, particularly for carbs, which can then increase insulin levels even more, which can lead to more carb cravings, creating a vicious cycle. Due to their insulin resistance, endomorphs process carbs poorly—and for these folks, excessive carbs will cause blood sugar spikes and crashes, leading to problematic spikes in the stress hormone cortisol and ultimately depleting their energy levels. Meanwhile, carbs that are consumed but not burned off for immediate energy get stored as body fat and glycogen.

This combination of factors makes endomorphs particularly prone to being leptin-resistant. Remember, leptin, often called the "satiety hormone," tells your brain that you have eaten enough food and that you have enough fat stored and it's okay to burn fat for fuel. If this signaling mechanism isn't working properly, you'll want to continue eating food, even if you've had enough, instead of using stored body fat for fuel.

As you've read on previous pages, body fat requires only a fraction of the calories that muscle does to sustain itself. So, having a greater proportion of body fat, as endomorphs do, translates into burning fewer calories per day. Simply put, high body fat = slow metabolism. This reality stinks and it creates another Catch-22 situation whereby having a higher percentage of body fat and a slower metabolism makes it harder to shed that body fat.

In addition, endomorphs often have high levels of the stress hormone cortisol, as a result of prolonged high insulin levels. But the effect can go the other way, too, because chronically elevated cortisol levels lead to increased insulin levels. It's an unfortunate round robin! Complicating matters, high cortisol levels promote the storage of body fat, especially in and around the belly. In other words, endomorphs often face a threatening triple whammy: leptin resistance, insulin resistance, and improperly regulated cortisol levels become a three-headed beast that can make weight control extra difficult. (For the record, exercise reduces cortisol levels and stabilizes insulin levels, but if you don't exercise enough and you continually feed your elevated insulin levels with carbs, the hormonal imbalance and your weight struggles will continue.)

I know this may sound like a whole lot of bad news, but there's plenty of hope because endomorphs do have the capacity to build more muscle, which will make all of these things better. Much. Better. With optimal eating habits and the right training format, endomorphs can give their bodies a higher muscle content, which can in turn ramp up their metabolic rate and improve their insulin sensitivity, making it easier to control their weight. The first thing that needs to change is the ratio of carbs in their diet (it needs to come down), perhaps with a reduction in calories, as well.

Take my client George, 53, a highly accomplished businessman, as an example. Naturally big-boned, he came to me with a soft belly and excess pounds that were exacerbated by years of globe-trotting travel, dining out, no exercise, and lots of stress, alcohol, and sugary snacks. The first thing we did was clean up his eating habits by drastically reducing his carb intake and focusing on smart food choices (lean protein, lots of veggies, healthy fats) at home and on the road.

We also got him into a workout program that involved 30 to 45 minutes of walking on a treadmill or stair-stepping machine at a brisk but sustainable pace five days per week; then, we eventually added three 1-hour weight-training sessions per week, sometimes with 15-minute HIIT sessions afterwards. He ended up working out five out of seven days per week—by doubling up with cardio and strength training, three times a week—so that he had two rest days each week. In eight months, he lost 36 pounds from his 6'1" frame and went from being unable to do a single push-up to doing sets of 40. Now, he can also do pull-ups and squats with 200-pound weights. *Amazing!* He also dropped multiple clothing sizes. It became a running joke that working with me cost him thousands of dollars in new clothes. A pretty great trade, if you ask me.

SLIMMING DOWN, SHAPING UP

For endomorphs who want to lose body fat and build lean muscle, a Paleo-style diet easily hits the right ratio of macronutrients. The Paleo diet is based on eating what the human body needed back in the Paleolithic era—I'm talking hunter-gatherer times, caveman days. The basic premise is high protein (38 percent of total calories), high fat (39 percent), and low carbs (23 percent). Lean protein would come from seafood and meat; fat would come from seeds, nuts, and meat sources. Grains, legumes, dairy products, soy, and refined sugar were simply not regular options in those days, so our Paleolithic predecessors didn't eat them.

I like a modified Paleo approach—one that includes legumes and healthy oils, in small doses—for endomorphs, and here's why: endomorphs struggle with carbs but digest protein and fat just fine; keeping protein intake high, especially when adding resistance training to the mix, ensures that muscle remains in top shape and is properly repaired. My suggested ratio of macronutrients for endomorphs is 40 percent protein, 40 percent fat, and 20 percent carbs. Avoid high-glycemic carbs (which increase blood sugar and insulin levels rapidly, in turn promoting fat accumulation, especially in the mid-section), sugary or refined foods, dairy products, and soy foods. (Note: if you're a vegetarian, you can have up to a 4-ounce serving of organic tofu or tempeh per day but don't go overboard with soy products.)

Because endomorphs tend to be insulin-resistant, it's best to consume carbs before and after your workouts—that's when your muscles really need them to fuel up and replenish glycogen stores. Otherwise, high-carb foods are quickly converted to blood sugar and can easily be stored as body fat. For the endomorph, it's best to think of carbs only to be used as "instant fuel." If you don't need them, don't have them. (FYI: This does not include vegetables or legumes; they get a free pass. I'm talking primarily about grains and fruit, to a lesser extent.)

Endomorphs who want to lose weight should keep their calories lower at first—usually between 1,300 and 1,500 calories initially. (To calculate your body's needs, use the BMR and TDEE formulas in Chapter Three). You can adjust this range, based on your rate of weight loss and your energy level. As a starting point, your macronutrient range should be 100 to 150 grams (400 to 600 calories) of protein, 40 to 60 grams (360 to 540 calories) of fat, and 60 to 80 grams (240 to 320 calories) of carbs.

Once you repair your hormone function and start burning more calories through exercise, this baseline calorie intake will be adjusted upward. Endomorphs (and other body types who have a history of crash dieting, starving, or malnourishing their bodies) frequently find success with an approach called "reverse dieting": this involves eating less and working out more initially then slowly increasing your calories and reducing your cardio workouts; this approach allows you to repair your metabolism and find the sweet spot where you can maintain a leaner physique, perform well at the gym, and stay healthy and energized. Endomorphs are much more diet-controlled than the other body types, so adjusting to this spot (physiologically and psychologically) may take a couple weeks. Be patient.

With this initial approach, here's what a week's worth of meals looks like:

SUNDAY

Breakfast: 3 whole eggs, scrambled with 1 cup chopped veggies (onions, mushrooms, spinach, zucchini) in 1 tablespoon coconut oil

Snack: 12 almonds, handful of carrot sticks

Lunch: 2 cups fresh chopped kale (or spinach), ½ cup sliced cherry tomatoes, ½ cup chopped cucumber, topped with 4 ounces grilled chicken breast, 1 tablespoon extra-virgin olive oil, 1–2 tablespoons balsamic vinegar; ½ cup cooked quinoa (if you'll be working out in the morning or early afternoon; otherwise add this to dinner)

Snack: 1 cup celery sticks with 2 tablespoons hummus

Dinner: 4 ounces grilled or broiled salmon served on 1 cup zucchini noodles sautéed in ½ tablespoon coconut oil, 1 cup roasted cauliflower

MONDAY

Breakfast: 2 slices cooked turkey bacon (chopped), scrambled with 3 egg whites and 1 cup spinach in ½ tablespoon coconut oil

Snack: 2 celery stalks spread with 1 tablespoon almond butter

Lunch: Swiss chard wraps, made with 3 ounces cooked ground turkey, ¼ cup black beans, ½ cup salsa, ½ large yellow bell pepper (chopped), divided between 2–3 large Swiss chard leaves

Snack: Protein shake, ½ cup raspberries

Dinner: 6 large grilled shrimp, 1 cup each grilled zucchini strips and grilled onion slices, drizzled with 1 tablespoon garlicky extra-virgin olive oil; ½ cup cooked quinoa (if you'll be working out in the morning or afternoon)

TUESDAY

Breakfast: 2 poached eggs with 1 cup spinach sautéed in 1 tablespoon coconut oil

Snack: 1 protein bar, ½ cup blueberries

Lunch: 1 cup gazpacho, topped with 1 tablespoon pumpkin seeds and a sprinkle of fresh basil; cooked 4-ounce turkey burger wrapped in lettuce leaf with sliced avocado and tomato

Snack: 1 small apple (sliced), topped with 1 tablespoon peanut butter, dash of cinnamon

Dinner: 4 ounces broiled chicken breast, 10 steamed asparagus spears, small side salad

WEDNESDAY

Breakfast: Morning parfait,* green juice*

Snack: Protein shake, ½ cup berries

Lunch: 4 ounces smoked wild salmon on 1 cup shredded fresh kale, with ¼ large carrot (grated), ½ cucumber (diced), 1 tablespoon extra-virgin olive oil, juice from ¼ lemon

Snack: 2 thin slices roasted turkey, wrapped around tomato slices

Dinner: 4 ounces broiled grass-fed flank steak, 1 cup zucchini noodles sautéed in 1 tablespoon grapeseed oil with ½ red pepper (sliced), ½ cup cooked quinoa (if afternoon workout)

THURSDAY

Breakfast: 2 omelet muffins*

Snack: 1 cup plain Greek or Icelandic yogurt, ½ cup strawberry slices

Lunch: 2 cups mixed greens with 1½ cups raw or cooked vegetables (such as broccoli, green beans, radishes), 4 ounces grilled chicken breast, 1 tablespoon extra-virgin olive oil, 1 tablespoon balsamic vinegar; ½ cup cooked brown rice (if you'll be working out in the late morning or early afternoon)

Snack: 2 tablespoons pumpkin seeds, 1 orange

Dinner: Fish tacos made with 4 ounces grilled or broiled mahi-mahi, ½ avocado (sliced), ½ cup salsa, two large lettuce leaves; 1 cup steamed broccoli on the side

FRIDAY

Breakfast: Butternut squash pancakes,* topped with ½ cup Icelandic vanilla yogurt, 1 tablespoon slivered almonds

Snack: 1 small pear with 1 tablespoon almond butter

Lunch: 1 cup lentil soup,* 3 ounces roasted turkey with 1 cup fresh spinach

Snack: 1 cup sugar snap peas with 2 tablespoons hummus

Dinner: 4 ounces grilled or broiled salmon, 1 cup roasted butternut squash, 10 asparagus spears, ½ cup cooked quinoa mixed with 1 tablespoon chopped pecans

SATURDAY

Breakfast: 2 poached eggs, topped with 1–2 tablespoons salsa and half an avocado (chopped), drizzled with 1 teaspoon extra-virgin olive oil, salt and pepper to taste

Snack: 1 protein bar

Lunch: 2 cups baby spinach with 4 ounces cooked grass-fed beef tenderloin (sliced thinly), ½ cup red pepper strips, ½ cup broccoli florets, 1 tablespoon extra-virgin olive oil

Snack: ½ cup fresh raspberries with 1 tablespoon chia seeds and 1 tablespoon walnuts

Dinner: 4 ounces chicken breast (cut into chunks), stir-fried with ½ cup chopped mushrooms, 1 cup broccoli florets, ¼ cup shredded carrots, ½ cup shredded cabbage, ¾ cup spinach; served on ½ cup cooked brown rice (if afternoon workout)

* Recipes included in Appendix B.

While consistency is important with your eating habits, you don't want your meals to become monotonous, nor do you want to force yourself to eat foods you don't like. But if you do have meals you especially enjoy and you are happy to eat frequently, I highly recommend preparing a week's worth at a time (then refrigerating or freezing them), so they're ready to have when you want them. This way, you can eliminate the stress of cooking or eating out too often. You can also trade a serving of any of the foods in the outlined meals and replace it with a food from the table below in the same category—

but be careful not to increase your carbs, in particular. Also, make sure you stick with the recommended serving size—don't just eyeball it, because it's easy to underestimate how much food you're serving yourself. Remember, too, that you should consume more protein and more carbs before and after your workouts.

CARBS	PROTEINS	FATS
sweet potatoes	chicken/turkey	nuts
Ezekiel bread	eggs/egg whites	seeds (pumpkin, chia, sprouted)
oats	fish	eggs
brown rice	broccoli/lentils/black beans	coconut oil (hot or cold)
quinoa	protein powder	olive oil (cold)

THE ENDOMORPH SLIM DOWN, SHAPE UP WORKOUT

When it comes to your workouts, your best bet is to focus initially on low- to moderate-intensity aerobic exercise such as walking briskly on a small incline on the treadmill three times a week for 30 to 45 minutes, in order to torch those fat stores your body has been stubbornly holding onto. Plus, building up cardiovascular endurance will allow you to boost your performance and stamina—and hence your motivation—on the calisthenics/strength-training regimen when you get to it. One strength-builder to add to your cardio regimen from the start: body-weight-based movements, such as lunges, squats, push-ups, and planks—basic, single-plane exercises without rotations. These will be hard at first, but your body will respond very well to this extra stimulation. If you're not new to exercise and you can already jog a mile without becoming short of breath, you can skip the "intro" phase and start with the strength training/HIIT phase (see Phase 3).

After your body becomes accustomed to the cardio regimen (say, in a week or two), you'll want to add strength training three times a week while keeping your brisk but steady cardio workouts constant. This two-step approach will help you burn body fat first and improve your blood pressure, blood sugar, and heart rate; then, you'll be able to maintain those health and conditioning gains while slowly building muscle, which will help you crank up your metabolic rate and burn more calories 24/7.

Weight training will then become a priority for shaping the body and continuously increasing muscle mass and metabolic function over time. That being said, daily brisk walks in the zone of 70 percent of your maximum heart rate (MHR) will readily and steadily burn calories, especially from fat, and keep your weight-loss journey primed for ongoing success.

So here's the plan:

PHASE 1 (WEEKS 1 TO 2):

At least three times per week walk briskly on a slight incline on a treadmill for 30 to 45 minutes. Your heart rate should be in the zone of 70 percent of your MHR. In addition, perform a series of push-ups (on your knees is fine), squats, planks, and side planks (these can be done with your knees on the floor if need be). Try to work up to doing 50 push-ups and squats, plus 1-minute planks and 30-second side planks, every other day. If doing more than 5 at a time is difficult at first, do 10 sets of 5 reps with breaks in between.

PHASE 2 (WEEKS 3 TO 4):

Increase the frequency of your cardio workouts to five times per week, at the same intensity and pace as the previous weeks. Do the body-weight-based strength-building moves (as above), two to three times per week before your cardio sessions.

PHASE 3 (AFTER 5 WEEKS):

Continue your cardio workouts five times per week and add the following strength-training workouts to your regimen three times per week. (First, warm up your muscles with a 5-minute stint on a cardio machine, doing burpees, or jumping rope.) Choose a weight where doing the desired number of repetitions (reps) feels difficult but not impossible on the first set. You'll find descriptions of all the exercises in Appendix A.

WORKOUT 1:

Do the following moves sequentially, including a 60-second break between each set.

3 sets of 1-minute Planks

3 sets of 8–12 Barbell Squats

2 sets of 20 Squat Jumps

3 sets of 10–15 Flat Bench Presses

2 sets of 15 Incline Dumbbell Presses

3 sets of 8 Deadlifts

3 sets of 15 Lat Pulldowns (wide grip)

3 sets of 10 Ab Wheel Rollouts

WORKOUT 2:

Do the following moves sequentially, including a 60-second break between each set.

3 sets of 12 seated Shoulder Presses with Dumbbells

3 sets of 15 Lateral Raises

3 sets of 15 Barbell Biceps Curls

3 sets of 8–10 Hammer Curls

2 sets of 20 Triceps Rope Pushdowns

3 sets of Push-Ups (as many as you can do at a time)

3 sets of 20 Knee Raises, followed immediately by 30 Back Extensions or Supermans

3 sets of 10 V-Ups, followed immediately by 20 Glute Kickbacks (with each leg)

WORKOUT 3:

Do the following moves sequentially, including a 60-second break between each set.

3 sets of 10 Romanian Deadlifts

2 sets of 20 Walking Lunges (add dumbbells if you need more of a challenge)

2 sets of 10 Burpees with Push-Ups

3 sets of 15 Incline Dumbbell Flies

3 sets of 8 45-degree Bent Rows (with free weights or a machine)

2 sets of 20 Lat Pulldowns (underhanded grip)

2 sets of 15 Dumbbell Biceps Curls

2 sets of 15 Triceps Kickbacks

2 sets of Triceps Dips (as many as you can do at a time)

2 sets of Planks (hold it as long as you can), immediately followed by Side Planks on both sides (hold each as long as you can)

When you're comfortable with the frequency of the cardio and strength-training workouts, add two sessions of HIIT each week—it's a great way to stimulate extra fat burning. But if you find that the HIIT leaves you sore and tired and unable to perform the weight training optimally, then you may want to cut back to one HIIT session per week or swap a HIIT workout for a lighter cardio session. Rest is incredibly important for muscle recovery, and you don't want to risk over-training, especially if you're in a calorie-cutting situation. So listen to your body and let it guide you.

BODY-WEIGHT HIIT WORKOUT:

To perform the following HIIT segment, all you need is your own body weight. Perform all the reps of each exercise without stopping, then immediately move on to the next exercise.

20 Squats

10 Push-Ups

30-second Plank, 30-second Side Plank on each side (for 1½ minutes total)

30 seconds of Mountain Climbers

20 Supermans

10 Burpees (without Push-Ups)

Take a 30-second break then repeat this sequence as many times as you can in 15 minutes.

• TROUBLESHOOTING TIPS •

IF YOUR WEIGHT is changing by more than two pounds per week in either direction after the first week or two, check your portions to make sure that you're not eating more or less than you think you are. (Get out the food scale and measuring cups and spoons, if need be.) If you're sure your portions are accurate and you're gaining too much weight, try cutting 10 to 20 percent from your food intake across the board. If you're losing more than two pounds per week, try adding 10 to 20 percent to your daily intake. It's important to keep the rate of your weight change in the healthy zone.

• • •

THE CREATING AND SHAPING MUSCLE PLAN

When I began working with Kate, 43, a business consultant in the LA area, she was healthy and fit but wanted to get stronger and shed some body fat. Her most pressing goal: she wanted to be able to do pull-ups. An endomorph with substantial muscle strength but also some extra padding on her figure, Kate had been following a mostly vegetarian—almost vegan—diet and doing cardio workouts twice a week and a HIIT-style boot-camp session once a week. She came to me with great lifestyle habits, but she wanted to do more for her body.

Because she was already doing cardio workouts regularly but no strength training, that's what we focused on from the get-go. We started her lifting weights with me twice per week, and I gave her a program for a third weight-lifting day that she could do on her own, as well as some guidance for daily low-intensity cardio. On the dietary front, we kept her on a vegetarian regimen but shifted her macronutrient ratio to 30 percent protein, 30 percent carbs, and 40 percent fat. To get there, we prioritized high-quality plant proteins such as tempeh, beans, legumes, quinoa, and nondairy yogurt and balanced them with good-quality carbs like zucchini, butternut squash noodles, and salads. She also timed the majority of her carbs around her workouts with high-fiber, low-glycemic choices to minimize the impact on her insulin levels.

She hadn't told her HIIT boot-camp group that she was training with me—and within weeks, they wanted to know her secret because they noticed she was trimming down and performing much better in the class. (She 'fessed up.) Within several months, Kate dropped 10 pounds and several inches from her physique and crushed her goals (she can even do a pull-up now). Now, she's setting new ones.

If you're trying to add muscle to your body without losing weight, it's important that you tweak your diet to support your goals. You can use the weight-loss plan, previously described, but add 200 to 300 calories per day to it, with an additional 25 grams of protein, 25 grams of carbs, and 10 grams of fat. Tread lightly on the calorie increase, though, because while endomorphs can add muscle quickly, they also can add body fat if they end up with a calorie surplus. Think of it this way: your diet can determine the size of your body, while exercise determines its shape—so you want to maintain the right synergy to achieve your goals.

What you really want to do is achieve a slow and steady "recomposition" of your body's fat-to-muscle ratio: by eating the right macronutrients at the right calorie level and working out in a strategic way, you'll maximize muscle sparing (maintenance) or muscle growth while keeping your fat-burning furnace turned on. Be sure to include protein and carbs in your meals or snacks before and after your workouts to help your muscles grow and recover properly.

As far as your workouts go, if you're new to exercise, start with Phases 1 and 2 on the endomorph weight-loss plan. After that, or if you've been exercising regularly (the way Kate was when we started working together), continue your cardio workouts five times per week (for 30 to 45 minutes at a time) and add the following strength-training workouts to your regimen three times per week to build muscle.

First, warm up with a 5-minute stint on a cardio machine, doing burpees, or jumping rope. For the moves that follow, choose a weight where doing the desired number of repetitions (reps) feels difficult but not impossible on the first set.

LEGS/CORE:

3 sets of 20 Glute Kickbacks (on each side)
3 sets of 15 Leg Presses (on a machine)
4 sets of 6–10 Barbell Squats
3 sets of 12 Hamstring Curls (on a machine)
2 sets of 15 Glute Bridges (with a barbell)
3 sets of 15 Incline Sit-Ups
2 sets of 20 Knee Raises (from a hanging position, if possible)

CHEST/BACK:

3 sets of 12–15 Incline Dumbbell Presses

3 sets of 6–10 Flat Bench Presses

4 sets of 8–12 Dumbbell Flies

3 sets of 10 Chest Dips (use a machine if you need to)

3 sets of 10 Bent Rows

3 sets of 12–15 Deadlifts

4 sets of 15 Lat Pulldowns (use a narrow grip handle)

3 sets of 8–10 One-Arm Dumbbell Rows (each side)

SHOULDERS/ARMS/CORE:

3 sets of 20 Lateral Raises

2 sets of 15 Shoulder Presses with Dumbbells

3 sets of 8–10 Shoulder Presses (on a machine)

3 sets of 10 Seated Biceps Curls, followed immediately by 10 Shoulder Presses with Dumbbells

2 sets of 20 Hammer Curls

3 sets of 10 Preacher Curls

3 sets of 20 Overhead Triceps Extensions

3 sets of 15 Triceps Rope Pushdowns

2 sets of 6–10 Straight Bar Pushdowns

3 sets of 30-second Mountain Climbers, followed immediately by 10 V-Ups

3 sets of 30-second Bicycles, followed immediately by 20 Supermans

3 sets of 1-minute Planks with Alternating Arm/Leg Lifts for 30 seconds

THE PAYOFFS

For many endomorphs, making the dietary changes in these plans is the most daunting aspect. But I assure you: once you start consuming more protein and trimming your carb intake, you'll grow accustomed to this approach very quickly—and you may even experience a substantial energy boost in the process. Many people do. If you're brand-spanking new to exercise, the workouts may seem challenging (on paper, at least). That's why I have newbies start with walking (something we all know how to do) and add to the program in a manageable fashion from there.

Stay attuned to your body every step of the way so you can tweak the program as needed. Also pay attention to physiological changes in your body, which are likely to come relatively quickly. In the short term, you'll get a rush from the boost in circulation and the release of feel-good endorphins that's very gratifying. Within several weeks, you'll probably notice considerable progress and gains in your muscle strength and stamina if you do these workouts consistently. Keep at it because before you know it, you'll start to see a difference in your physique: your body will likely become tighter and firmer, and you'll start to notice greater muscle definition, too. Appreciate and celebrate these changes because they're signs that you're giving your body the fuel and the stimulation it needs to become its best self yet.

HYBRID BODY TYPES

QUITE OFTEN, PEOPLE DON'T FALL EXCLUSIVELY INTO ONE body type category or another. Many of us are basically mixed breeds—and may even have certain influences more prominently within the same family. A woman or man will likely have predominant traits of one body type but with significant crossover influences from another body type. The two most common hybrids are a meso-endomorph—with a curvaceous and athletic build (like model Elizabeth Hurley and actress Minnie Driver, actors Steve Howey and Henry Cavill)—and an ecto-mesomorph—with a coveted "V" shape for a man's body (think Hugh Jackman and Christian Bale) and long, lean limbs but with muscular definition for a woman's body (like professional volleyball player/sports announcer Gabrielle Reece or Victoria's Secret top model Candice Swanepoel).

Each hybrid has its own blend of physical attributes and responses to dietary and physical training regimens. With the right adjustments, every person with a mixed body type can maximize his or her inherent assets, as you'll see.

CURVY AND MUSCULAR: THE MESO-ENDOMORPH

The meso-endomorph tends to have a thick midsection and a noticeably strong upper body (think: wide shoulders, thick chest, muscular arms), as well as larger buttocks and legs. If the endomorph side is more dominant, endo-mesomorphs may retain a substantial amount of water, especially when their diets are suboptimal (in this case, even when muscle is present and firm, the outer layers may be masked by a combination of fat and water). Both men and women with this body type have a striking appearance in that they look strong, maybe even somewhat boxy, with obvious muscle size and tone. These folks really excel at high-intensity sports and physical activities involving strength and power because they have a mix of high amounts of type 2 (fast-twitch) muscle fibers but also more athleticism and endurance than a pure endomorph does. Given this, it's not surprising that research has found meso-endomorphs tend to be the primary body type of young male soccer goalkeepers, adult male tennis players, elite female handball players and water polo players (especially centers), and elite baseball players. This type also builds and retains muscle very well, excellent qualities for bodybuilding and powerlifting.

Depending on the person's diet, muscle and fat can be easily added to his or her meso-endo physique (whether it's wanted or not). That's why if you're a meso-endomorph and you want to trim fat from your body, it's wise to time your carbohydrate consumption around your workouts. For endo-mesomorphs who want to change their body, diet is the most important variable. These folks often inherit the endomorph tendency to be somewhat insulin resistant, which means they can struggle with handling high carb loads. This body type often holds onto excess water and glycogen stores so an easy way to shed body fat and water is to "carb cycle": one day, you might have a low carb intake with a higher intake of protein and fat; the next day, you might consume moderate amounts of carbs as well as moderate amounts of protein and fat.

Based on their weight, endo-mesomorphs may have three to six days' worth of glycogen stores built up, which makes these folks resistant to fat-burning by nature. Because they have so much glycogen in reserve, their bodies don't turn to stored fat as a source of fuel. So it's important to jump-start the fat-burning process, and carb cycling is a great way to do that. Carbs can carry up to three times their weight in water, so if you're eating and storing carbs as glycogen, you can end up with extra "weight" on you that can be easily shed with a simple macronutrient switch.

Some easy shortcuts to help you get to the right prize:

+ If fat loss is your main goal, stick to a pure endomorph diet (see page 80) and keep your carbs low (20 percent of your daily calories) consistently; if you end up feeling depleted and need a "boost" day with higher carbs because of your workouts, have a treat meal with double the portion of carbs, two to three times per week. Otherwise, stick with a meal plan that consists of 40 percent protein, 40 percent fat, and 20 percent carbs (example: a breakfast of 3 whole eggs, scrambled with 1 cup chopped veggies in 1 tablespoon coconut oil).
+ If your goal is to shed body fat while gaining muscle, follow the endomorph diet (20 percent carbs) on your non-strength-training days and the basic mesomorph diet (30 percent carbs, 35 percent protein, 35 percent fat; see page 63) on your weight-lifting days. Think of this as a simple hack to feed your muscles when they need it without making you store fat when they don't. Here's what two consecutive days of meals might look like with this approach:

NON-STRENGTH-TRAINING DAY:

Breakfast: 3 whole eggs, scrambled with 1 cup chopped veggies (onions, mushrooms, spinach, zucchini) in 1 tablespoon coconut oil

Snack: 12 almonds, handful of carrot sticks

Lunch: 2 cups fresh chopped kale (or spinach), ½ cup sliced cherry tomatoes, ½ cup chopped cucumber, topped with 4 ounces grilled chicken breast, 1 tablespoon extra-virgin olive oil, balsamic vinegar; ½ cup cooked quinoa (if you'll be working out in the morning or early afternoon; otherwise add this to dinner)

Snack: 1 cup celery sticks with 2 tablespoons hummus

Dinner: 4 ounces grilled or broiled salmon served on 1 cup zucchini noodles sautéed in ½ tablespoon coconut oil, 1 cup roasted cauliflower

STRENGTH-TRAINING DAY:

Breakfast: 1 cup cooked oatmeal topped with ½ cup blueberries, 1 tablespoon chopped walnuts, ½ tablespoon chia seeds, ¼ teaspoon cinnamon; hardboiled egg

Snack: 1 protein bar, ½ cup melon chunks

Lunch: Salad with lots of leafy greens, cut-up beets, apple slices, ½ cup chickpeas, 1 tablespoon vinaigrette, 4 ounces grilled chicken

Snack: ½ cup roasted chickpeas, 12 almonds

Dinner: 4 ounces roasted rainbow trout, ½ cup cooked quinoa, 2 cups shaved zucchini, summer squash, radish, and carrot, mixed with chopped dill, 1 teaspoon extra-virgin olive oil, ½ teaspoon rice wine vinegar

Consider my client Emma, 28, a fitness model with a naturally athletic but slightly boxy figure. Because she wants to get into acting, she decided to focus on making her body more slender while maintaining its strength. To make that happen, we manipulated her macronutrient intake, taking down her protein and carbs and adding a bit more fat, and changed her cardio workouts to more low intensity than her usual four-times-per-week HIIT regimen. Meanwhile, we kept her strength-training workouts to three times per week for 45 minutes at a time, so she could preserve her strength and muscle mass but help it become leaner and drop body fat in a controlled fashion. Within four months, Emma went from carrying 160 pounds on her 5'7" figure to 145 pounds, and gained a leaner but still curvy and strong appearance. Basically, she optimized her body's natural constitution by tweaking her diet and exercise approach, to give her a different "look" than she was used to. She truly appreciated the difference.

Meanwhile, on the exercise front, it's best to incorporate a mix of HIIT and low-intensity cardio sessions into your regimen with a greater focus on high-rep (12 to 20 reps) resistance training with moderately heavy weights; this approach will help you maximize your results and create a tight, toned physique. To address "trouble spots" (areas, really), I recommend doubling down by doing isolation exercises (such as glute kickbacks, biceps curls, triceps extensions, lateral raises, or other movements that target just one muscle that you want to define more). While endo-mesomorphs may tire and lose strength in the gym as a session goes on, they can generally handle more training than some other body types can since endo-mesos have more muscle mass and ample glycogen stores (think of this as a hidden supply of fuel for your muscles).

The optimal approach for these folks is to follow the mesomorph muscle-building exercise regimen (see page 69), but to increase the number of reps by about 20 percent (so instead of doing 10 Flat Bench Presses on the meso plan, you'd do 12 reps; instead of doing 20 Dumbbell Flies, you'd do 24), including burnout sets or supersets on the last exercise. This means you'll do weight training three to four times per week; as with other plans, you'll want to choose a weight where doing the desired number of reps feels difficult but not impossible on the first set.

Going overboard with cardio workouts can backfire for endo-mesomorphs. You may find that if you're training hard, doing higher reps and a greater intensity (or volume) of strength training, *and* doing too much cardio, you end up feeling perpetually hungry. The problem is, if you burn 400 calories per day with running or cycling but you consume an extra 600 calories throughout the day as a result, the net result is that you're adding calories, rather than burning more. *That's not what you want!* The approach I find to be most successful with my endo-mesomorph clients is doing low-intensity cardio for 30 to 45 minutes three times per week to burn body fat and build or maintain heart health, combined with 15 to 20 minutes of HIIT workouts two or three times per week. At the gym, I see a lot of endo-mesomorphs who are muscly but soft, spending an hour or more every day on the exercise bike or elliptical trainer without doing any weight workouts. Trust me, this is not going to change their bodies the way many of them want it to.

If appetite stimulation and overeating are problems, I have my endo-mesomorph clients separate their cardio workout days (avoid doing them consecutively, in other words). I know: life is busy, so if you have to double up with a strength-training workout and a cardio workout on the same day, that's fine. Just don't "double-double"—meaning, don't do a particularly intense strength-training workout and a super-intense cardio workout on the same day and don't double up two days in a row. Your body needs sufficient rest and recovery to optimize your hormone levels and transform into a tighter, more toned version of itself.

LONG AND STRONG: THE ECTO-MESOMORPH PHYSIQUE

By contrast, someone with an ecto-mesomorph physique may look lean and athletic (think swimmer's build) and excel at activities involving power and endurance. Interestingly, research has found that ecto-mesomorphs have high-level performance in elite bouldering (climbing), surfing, and triathlons. My brother-in-law, Thomas Rivers Puzey, is one of the purest ecto-mesos I have ever seen (even more so than me!). A world-class fitness model, runner, and Ironman, Thomas, 34, can run with some of the fastest people in the world, even though he was always 15 to 20 pounds heavier than his competitors. The truth is, he looks like a giant, with much more muscle than pure ectomorphs have. At one point, Thomas was purposefully losing weight and he ended up in a starved state (we called him *The Machinist* after the emaciated Christian Bale character in the 2004 movie), but even then, he couldn't turn his body into a pure ectomorph because he still had muscle, a V-shaped torso, and strong bones. Instead, he's the perfect hybrid, an endurance/muscular crossover fitness model and athlete. Lucky guy. Thomas ran the 2017 Boston Marathon in 2:18, winning 16th place overall. Conversely, he won his first triathlon and qualified for the world Kona Ironman his very first year after only months of training—that's unheard of. While he doesn't have incredible speed, he has the leg and upper body power that his competitors didn't, thanks to insanely hard work and 15 years of competitive running that helped him build world-class endurance.

Ecto-mesomorphs can thrive on a simple, balanced food plan, with a diet comprised of almost exactly one-third each of protein, carbs, and fats. They can digest and process all macronutrients well and have fast metabolisms. If extra fat does creep onto their bods, there's a good chance it will be on the midsection (as in the belly or buttocks), in which case they may want to ramp up protein intake and dial down carb consumption. Take me, for example: as a highly active ecto-mesomorph, I consume about 3,000 calories per day, and it's pretty close to 250 grams of protein, 250 grams of carbs, and 100 grams of fat. At 6' and 200 pounds, I have about 9 percent body fat—and this nutritional breakdown helps me maintain my body and my active lifestyle. I lift weights four days a week and get cardio workouts in two or three days per week in fun ways by playing with my kids, going to the beach, rock climbing, or doing HIIT hill sprints. This amounts to about an hour a day of working out, with a full rest day or even two each week. If I want to get super lean for an event, a photo session, or another reason, I will increase my protein intake (to 40 percent of my daily calories) and reduce my carbs slightly and add in a little more cardio. If I want to add muscle, I'll add a few hundred calories of protein (going up to 35 percent) and carbs (going up to 45 percent) and reduce my fat intake (to 20 percent). In other words, there's some wiggle room in the optimal nutritional approach for ecto-mesos, depending on their goals.

With this macronutrient ratio, breakfast could be 1 cup cooked oatmeal, topped with 1 tablespoon chopped walnuts, ½ cup blueberries, ½ tablespoon chia seeds, with ½ scoop protein powder. Lunch might consist of 1 cup black bean soup and ½ turkey sandwich (3 ounces roasted turkey, 1 tablespoon hummus, 1 slice tomato, 2 avocado slices, on 1 slice Ezekiel bread). Dinner could be 4–6 ounces grilled or broiled salmon, 1 baked sweet potato, and 12 steamed asparagus spears. Snacks might include a hardboiled egg and an apple, a cup of cottage cheese or Greek yogurt with berries, or a protein bar. (For the sake of simplicity, you can use the weight-loss mesomorph diet in Chapter Five as a guide, adding a smidgen more carbs.)

Since having an ecto-mesomorph body type allows you to build muscle quickly, your fitness regimen will depend on what your goal is: if you want to develop a lean and toned look without building visually prominent muscles, your best bet is to stick with steady-state, endurance cardio workouts (such as brisk walking or light jogging for 30 minutes) and plyometric strength training instead of high reps and heavy weights (train like a mesomorph, in other words; see workout in Chapter Five). On the other hand, if you want to develop impressive muscles, you'd be better off going with HIIT circuits (such as burpees, squats, jumping jacks, push-ups, and mountain climbers) in the 8 to 15 rep range; in this case, you'll want to aim for muscle failure, not just fatigue.

OPPOSING QUALITIES: THE ECTO-ENDOMORPH PHYSIQUE

Given that ectomorphs and endomorphs are at opposite ends of the somatotype spectrum, this hybrid type may seem to be impossible—but it's a modern phenomenon, which is why I'm including it here. Basically, an ecto-endomorph has the musculoskeletal system of an ectomorph but the person has lost his or her way in terms of diet and physical activity for so long or so drastically that his or her endocrine (hormonal) system has gone off course, veering toward insulin resistance. In other words, endomorphic properties of softness, insulin resistance, and fatigue have greatly changed the person's body, thus corrupting his or her natural ectomorph status. Depending on the level of change that has occurred, the ecto-endomorph still may be slim-limbed, but with larger fat stores around the belly, thighs, butt, and chest. If the changes have become more entrenched and penetrated the body more deeply, the person may look soft and bloated all over, due to hidden inflammation and water retention; in this case, this is almost like the person's internal systems are screaming, *This is not what we were meant to do!*

Either way, the challenge for these folks is to unmask their inner ectomorphs. Doing this requires dropping excess pounds (including body fat and water weight), optimizing their hormone levels, and eventually adding muscle. To get there, it's important to follow a strict endomorph weight-loss diet (see page 80) with low carbs (20 percent), 40 percent protein, and 40 percent fat; once the weight loss is significant (once you drop below 15 percent body fat, which would bring you back to more of an ectomorph physique), you can slowly add carbs back to see if you still feel energized and upbeat, which are signs that your body is back on track (and no longer flirting with insulin resistance), and can keep off the weight you've lost.

While eating like an endomorph, it's best if you start training like an ectomorph with heavy resistance training (including compound movements)—mostly keeping reps in the 8 to 12 range, with occasional 5-rep sets and 20-rep sets to the point of burnout—but with the low-intensity cardio workouts from the endomorph plan. Confused? Don't sweat it. Here's what this approach would look like:

LEGS/ABS DAY:

5 sets of 12 Weighted Squats

3 sets of 12 Romanian Deadlifts

3 sets of 20 Squat Jumps

3 sets of 12 Walking Lunges with dumbbells

3 sets of 10 Leg Presses (on a weight machine)

3 sets of Planks (holding each one as long as you can)

3 sets of Side Planks (holding each one as long as you can on each side)

3 sets of 15 V-Ups, immediately followed by 20 Supermans

CHEST/BACK DAY:

5 sets of 8–12 Incline Bench Presses

3 sets of 10 Flat Bench Presses with dumbbells

3 sets of 12 Dumbbell Pec Flies

3 sets of 12 Dips (use a machine that assists)

3 sets of Push-Ups to the point of failure

5 sets of 5–12 Lat Pulldowns (start light weight and high reps, add weight each set)

4 sets of 6–10 Bent Rows

4 sets of 8 Deadlifts

3 sets of 6–8 One-Arm Dumbbell Rows

SHOULDERS/ARMS DAY:

3 sets of 6–10 Shoulder Presses with Dumbbells

3 sets of 20 Lateral Raises

3 sets of 10 Front Dumbbell Raises

3 sets of 15 seated Military Presses on a Smith machine

With the exercises that follow, you'll want to do 10–15 reps per set, with 3-second negatives: this means slowing down the lowering or downward part of the lift—the eccentric phase, which is what causes the muscles to adapt and get stronger—to 3 seconds.

3 sets of alternating Standing Barbell Curls and Skull Crushers

3 sets of alternating Dumbbell Biceps Curls and Triceps Rope Pushdowns

3 sets of alternating Hammer Curls and Triceps Dips

As for cardio, focus on low-intensity aerobic exercise such as walking briskly on a slight incline on the treadmill three times a week for 30 to 45 minutes, in order to torch the fat stores your body has been stubbornly holding onto. Your heart rate should be in the zone of 70 percent of your MHR. When your physique has returned to a thinner ectomorph frame (woo-hoo!), even if it's still a little bit soft, you can focus on working to add muscle mass at a higher rate, using the ectomorph muscle-building workouts (see page 50) and the 40-40-20 ratio of carbs-protein-fat.

When I started working with Jeff, a successful Hollywood talent manager in his mid-40s, his body was soft, with very little strength, ample belly fat, and "man boobs" despite having slender limbs and bones. In other words, Jeff was an ectomorph who had let himself go and had become an ecto-endomorph. We put him on an endomorph eating plan (low carbs and only pre- and post-workout) until we got his body fat down from 20 percent to 14 percent, and we started an ectomorph-style training regimen with heavy resistance training (previously, he had been doing only cardio). After four months with this program, he lost 12 pounds of body fat and added some lean muscle. At that point, we began adding carbs back to his diet (in increments of 10 percent) while increasing his workouts. It's been a year since we started working together and he looks amazingly different—now, he is down to 10 percent body fat and has killer abs! The endomorph qualities are gone.

THE PAYOFFS

As you've seen, if you have a hybrid body type, that doesn't mean you've slipped through the cracks with the somatotype approach to maximizing your body type. *On the contrary!* It means you can borrow the diet and exercise strategies from two different body type plans in order to customize an approach that suits your body's needs and tendencies. I do this on a regular basis with my clients and they achieve incredible results. You will, too. Within weeks of following the hybrid plan that's right for you, you'll start slimming down, shaping up, and gaining greater muscle tightness, tone, or definition. And because you'll be mixing and matching approaches from different body-type plans to achieve *your* personal goals, you'll learn how to continuously tweak your diet and exercise habits in ways that will work for you in the long haul. That's a win-win outcome if ever there was one!

BUILDING MENTAL FITNESS

L ET'S FACE IT: WHEN IT COMES TO GETTING FIT (OR FITTER) OR
losing weight (or body fat), your mind can be your biggest
ally, or your worst foe. That's why it's smart to occasionally hit
the pause button and take your mental pulse: When you think
about your body, its state, shape, and capabilities, does your inner voice sound like it's coming from a kind, supportive coach or
a mean, abusive taskmaster? The answer matters because your
mind is your most powerful muscle, which means you can either
flex it to boost your motivation and perseverance or clench it
to resist or sabotage your own efforts. To make the right choice
(the latter one, in case you had any doubt), it's essential to have
a clear sense of why you've set a particular goal for yourself and

to remind yourself of the answers on a regular basis to help you stay on course and go the distance.

So go ahead and ask yourself, *What do I want to achieve? Why do I really want this?* And *How badly do I really want it?* The next step is to visualize achieving what you're striving for: picture yourself slipping into the strong, fit, toned body you want, and imagine how you'd look, feel, and move. Remember and revisit that image often to keep what you're striving for in the front of your mind.

If you want to make lifestyle changes that last and have the mental motivation to keep doing what you're doing, it's crucial to bring your head into the equation in myriad ways. Otherwise, you won't be mentally invested in the diet and exercise changes you're trying to make. The truth is, my clients who make the most progress have a hefty dose of self-motivation and self-discipline—mental fortitude—and you need these key ingredients, too. Even the best in-person workouts with me three or four times per week won't lead to optimal results if the other days are misused with excessive lounging on the couch, channel surfing, and junk-food orgies. So you really need to build mental fitness in tandem with physical fitness. One without the other isn't all that helpful, but the two together create a positive synergy in which one reinforces the other.

Here are essential ways to set that critical process in motion:

CREATE A **TYPE** GOAL. Unless you wanted to hit the road for the sheer thrill of it, you wouldn't get in your car and drive somewhere without a destination in mind. The same should be true of altering your diet and exercise habits. To make the journey as efficient and enjoyable as possible, you'll want to give yourself a physical and mental playbook so that your mind and your muscles can work together and support each other. To create that reciprocal positive connection, the best way to frame your goals is with the TYPE system. That means making them

T: Timely and time-based with a deadline to keep you motivated and on track

Y: You-centered, as in having a personally meaningful, specific target so you'll know what you're working toward

P: Plausible, as in realistic and attainable with action-oriented steps

E: Energizing so that your plan feels continuously fresh and you feel motivated to keep striving for the results you want.

To make this more relatable, let's break it down in . . . slo-mo:

T is for timely because if you aren't working with a specific timetable, you'll have no way to set your long- and short-term goals, calculate the right numbers for your diet or workouts, or keep various endpoints in mind. Leave the time-frame for losing weight or getting fitter open-ended and time is likely to slip away from you—and so will your goals. So set your sights on what you want to achieve and in what time period, with intermediate (or, stepping-stone) goals along the way.

Y is for you-centered because really this plan is all about you. This entire book is about learning to eat and exercise right for *your* body type—but it's up to *you* to set specific goals for yourself. You aren't competing against a friend or another group. This is about you creating the best version of yourself, developing a better understanding of yourself, and showing yourself some serious love by taking good care of yourself. So set a personally meaningful goal (or two) that you can work toward—and hold yourself accountable to doing what it takes to get to that prize. This way you'll be *much* more likely to achieve it and you can be proud of yourself.

P is for plausible because if your goal isn't realistic or attainable, you're not likely to reach it. So don't expect to develop your dream body in a week (or two or three). Think about what's realistic for you to achieve in a given span of time and frame your goals accordingly. If you want to lose 10 pounds, aim to shed 1 to 2 pounds per week and build your time line from there. Do the same thing if you want to be able to bench-press a specific amount of weight or run a certain distance. Once you achieve your goals, you can continue to set new ones that are outside your current comfort zone and expand your capabilities from there.

E is for energizing because you need goals and a plan that make you feel consistently excited and motivated to pursue them. Otherwise, your plan can start to feel basic or stale and you might start giving a half-baked effort. That's the opposite of what you want to happen! So make an effort to keep your plan lively, appealing, and inspiring so you'll want to keep chasing your goals.

This approach to setting goals works—and it works well. It lets you cover the bases of having key metrics—such as a measurable, realistic goal and a time frame to complete it in—and it forces you to make your goals personal and self-affirming. By way of example, consider actor Steve Howey, who wanted to get "as jacked as possible" for Season 7 of *Shameless*. It was a worthy goal but kind of vague so we broke it down into the specifics of how he would need to shed some weight and body fat first, then build up muscle to achieve a body recomposition for his endo-mesomorph body type. We turned it into a TYPE goal by making it timely (we had a year to work with until Season 7 filmed), keeping the plan centered on Steve's goals, making it plausible (by breaking the big goal into smaller ones and adjusting his macronutrient intake and workout approach accordingly), and making it energizing by celebrating the small victories along the way (like five-pound weight-loss milestones, new personal records with weight-lifting, and so on). It worked: he went from 242 pounds and 22 percent body fat to 220 with 10 percent body fat and killer

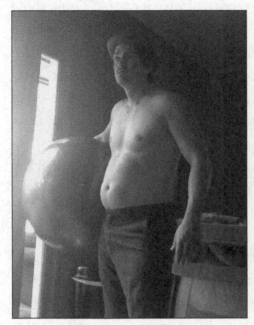 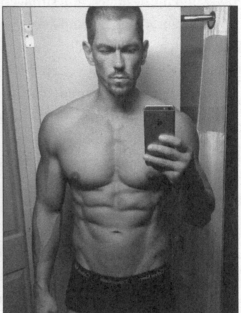

abs. *Want proof?* Check out the difference in how he looks on *Shameless* before Season 7 and after, when he truly does look jacked and ripped.

The TYPE model works because it is based on both *what* you want to accomplish and *why* you want it. In this book, I am providing you with all the *how*'s you'll need to transform your diet and your workouts in order to transform your body. Now it's time to get inside your head and transform your attitude in key ways. The following mental tips, tricks, and strategies will help you keep your physical and psychological energy and motivation high, as you strive for the prize you've set your sights on.

Run toward the positive, not away from the negative. Picture the results of what you're working to achieve and forget about the feelings and habits you're trying to ditch. Imagine what it would feel like to transform your body into the healthiest and strongest version of what it can be. Think about how vibrant, powerful, and sexy you'd feel, how you'd present yourself to the world, how you'd walk, run, or dance. As they're working toward body-enhancing goals, people often think about what they're trying to get away from (perhaps feeling tired, sluggish, depressed, insecure, or some other bummer of a feeling). But think about it: that's kind of like running away from a mugger while looking over your shoulder—it makes you likely to trip and fall. It's much more productive to envision your end goal and then run full-steam ahead toward it. Chase the image of what you want and you'll get to it so much faster.

Rewrite your internal script. Instead of just silencing the negative chatter in your head—you know, the voice that tells you that you aren't fit enough or strong enough to do a Tough Mudder race, a triathlon, or whatever physical event you want to do—replace that hyper-critical inner voice with one that takes a more positive view. Remind yourself of a time when you performed at your absolute best, whether it was while playing a particular sport, giving a presentation at work, or doing something else. Create a mantra that helps trigger those feelings of complete confidence and operating in the optimal performance zone. It doesn't have to be complicated; it can be something as simple as "I've got this!" or "I can do this!" Changing the way you think and talk (to yourself) about your physical capabilities can help you get the results you want. Want proof? Research suggests that perceived fitness (a person's belief about his or her level of physical fitness) is a stronger predictor of the psychological benefits and improvements in physical functioning that stem from exercise than the person's aerobic fitness level.

Embrace the right motivation. In a nutshell, the optimal form of motivation is intrinsic motivation (which comes from inside you and is long lasting) rather than extrinsic motivation (which comes from outside you and has an expiration date). Don't get me wrong: sometimes an external source of motivation (such as wanting to look good for a reunion or a wedding or to win a medal in a competition) can get you into a healthier lifestyle, but what happens after the motivating event has passed? It's not going to inspire you to sustain your lifestyle changes for the long run, that's for sure. On the other hand, internal motivation (which can stem from having a personally meaningful goal, enjoying the process or activity itself, and/or feeling gratified by your progress) can. So dig deep and find a sustainable, personally meaningful reason why you want to make these changes for the duration, why you want to be your healthiest, strongest, best self. Maybe it's to improve your health, have more energy, or be able to dance at your (future) child's wedding. There's no "right" answer. Whatever it is, the *why* behind your motivation is what really matters, so name it, embrace it, write it down, then integrate it into your TYPE goal. Keep it close to your heart and mind, and think of it whenever sticking to your diet or workouts feels especially tough. Think of this as your way to continuously light your own fire.

For example, I *want* and *need* to be healthy for my kids, and I want to be around to know my grandkids. For someone else, getting fit may be driven by a desire for greater internal confidence or a desire to overcome negative body image issues. For others, a passion for having a soul-enriching adventure—such as hiking a mountain in Nepal, going helicopter skiing, or doing a triathlon—may be the driving force. I work with a lot of men and women who are on the cusp of turning 40 or 50 and they decide they want to build their "best body ever": I'm happy to report that I have seen this desire come to fruition many times, as people develop impressive ab muscles or learn to do a pull-up for the first time at 40 and 50. The secrets to their success: creating a TYPE goal and then working hard to achieve it.

Actress Danielle Fishel came to me because her fiancé, writer-comedian-producer Jensen Karp, had seen great results from training with me. He had a very specific time-frame, goal, and idea in mind that we actually framed as a "challenge" called Buff Season for his podcast *Get Up on This*. Danielle's motivation started with a wedding date and a body shape and weight she wanted to have for her special day. As we started working together and got to know each other, it became clear that her motivation went even deeper, that she wanted to feel strong and full of energy for the big day and beyond. With her goals in mind, she came to every workout with a positive attitude and lots of energy—and she made progress every single week. Because she is a mesomorph, Danielle develops muscle and strength quickly, but it was her dedication, commitment, and continuous motivation that got her to her goals.

Celebrate the small mind-body gains. As you're working toward your ultimate goal, appreciate how much better you already feel in different areas of your life. Are you sleeping better? Do you have greater mental clarity and focus? More energy? Less pain? Is your skin glowing? Do you look healthier or more vibrant? A 2018 study from Virginia Commonwealth University found that men who did a single high-intensity interval workout on a stationary bicycle had significant improvements in their executive function (a set of cognitive skills involving the ability to plan, focus attention, remember instructions, and multitask successfully) immediately afterward. A study from the University of South Carolina found that after previously sedentary women engaged in a single 54-minute session of moderate exercise, they slept better and had fewer awakenings during the night. *Those are small victories right there!* By tuning into the more short-term benefits of the lifestyle changes you've made, you'll have strong incentive to continue the great work.

Picture yourself killing it. Believe it or not, visualizing yourself lifting weights, running faster, or climbing to a high peak with perfect form can help you achieve the real deal in actual life. The reason: "Visualization establishes a mental blueprint for sport skills and tactical ploys," as sport psychologists Costas Karageorghis and Peter Terry note in their book *Inside Sport Psychology*. Let's say you visualize yourself doing biceps curls: electrical activity can actually be detected in the biceps muscles (on electromyographical recordings) even without your doing any physical movement; this means that during mental rehearsals, the appropriate muscles are primed for subsequent action, which can lead to improvements in actual performance when the time comes. "When you practice mentally, your muscles are to some extent rehearsing the movement," Karageorghis and Terry explain. Sport psychologists even have an acronym for this phenomenon—WYSIWYG (for *What You See Is What You Get*). So go ahead and imagine yourself rocking your performance in the weight room, on the trail, or on the climbing wall, using as many senses as you can; the visual rehearsal will serve you well once you get to the workout itself.

Bargain with yourself. We all have our off days when we just don't feel like doing much. Rather than ditching your workout entirely, it's better to make a deal with yourself to show up and do whatever you'd planned to do for 10 minutes. Whether it's lifting weights, running, cycling, or something else, swing into action for 10 minutes and heed this rule: if you really want to quit after 10 minutes, give yourself permission to call it quits or pull the escape hatch. Even if you don't perform at your best, exercising for 10 minutes is better than bagging a workout entirely. But chances are, once your body gets into motion and you feel the endorphins start to kick in after 10 minutes, you'll be able to bargain with yourself to give it another 10 or 20 minutes and before you know it, you might just eke out a full workout.

Stay accountable to yourself. Striving for a goal without keeping yourself accountable to it is like taking a road trip to somewhere you've never been without using a map or GPS, or tracking your mileage or landmarks along the way. *Is it theoretically possible to get to your desired destination?* Sure, but you may get lost en route or take some unexpected (or unwanted) detours. Then again, you might not arrive where you wanted to at all. The reality is, the journey to greater fitness will go more quickly, efficiently, safely, and easily if you record your workouts (including the amount of weight you're lifting, the number of reps you're doing, and other important details) and monitor your progress in a journal, on an app, or somewhere else, noting key milestones along the way. Doing this can help with troubleshooting because you can see patterns between your performance and your lifestyle habits (whether you ate or slept well or took time to relax before you worked out, for example).

Here's an example from my own workout log (page 115), followed by a blank journal page you can copy and use for yourself.

At least on a monthly basis, check your objective numbers (for weights, reps, your body weight or measurements) to gauge your progress. The reason: numbers don't lie. You live in your body day after day so it's easy to be blind to incremental changes in your physique, but seeing a record of measurable numerical improvements will make you realize how far you've come—and it can give you a *huge* mental and motivational incentive to keep doing what you're doing. Sharing your goals and progress with friends and family members also can help you stay true to your cause: just be sure to share only with people you trust to build you up or support you—and who will be honest with you if you're going off track or overdoing it.

Accept your feelings. Listen, bad moods happen. Some days, work sucks. People cut you off on the freeway. You have a fight with your partner or a family member. You don't meet your workout goal. I get it: you're human. First of all, welcome to the club—I'm a member, too! We're all in this thing called "life" together, and it can feel liberating to acknowledge that it's okay to have off days or feel anxious or flail. It opens you up to being teachable

EXERCISE	WEIGHT	SETS	REPS	NOTES
Bench Press	245	3	10	Got first 2 sets, only 6 reps on the 3rd.
Incline DB Press	100	3	12	Got all 3, did burnout sets to failure with 30s after.
Pushups		3	Failure	22, 18, 5
Wide-Grip Pullups		5	Failure	25, 17, 14, 11, 8
Deadlifts	405	5	5	All done.
Bent Rows	225	3	12	All done
Incline Fly/Rear Fly supersets	20	3	15 of each	Did all back to back; burnouts for 30 sec.
Cable Crossovers	100	3	20	All done
Low-cable Rows	200	3	8	All done
Cardio	Finished with 15 mins treadmill HIIT.			
How I Felt Afterward	Overall good workout. Felt a little tired so didn't go as long or hard on the HIIT but still crushed it all in 65 mins total.			

Now, it's your turn:

EXERCISE	WEIGHT	SETS	REPS	NOTES
Cardio				
How I Felt Afterward				

and humble, attributes that you need for physical and psychological growth. So do the best you can on any given day and realize that you won't be able to give 100 percent every single day—and that's all right. My motto is: it's always better to do *something*, even if it's hard, than nothing.

There's no substitute for working hard and taking pride in that. When you show up for yourself, push through, and make things happen when life feels especially tough, you won't regret it. Even if you do a shorter-than-usual workout or give a 70 percent effort, you're still doing yourself a solid by doing something. Similarly, if your best dietary intentions go off the rails at a meal, cut yourself some slack and get back on track for the rest of the day and the next day. Repeat after me: *I am human.* Perfection isn't the goal (spoiler alert: it doesn't even exist) so do the best you can, and strive to make improvements when you realize you're not at the top of your game.

Get a grip on your moods. Exercise is one of the most effective mood managers on the planet so don't be surprised if you feel better after working up a sweat or pushing your physical limits. But if you still feel down, anxious, or otherwise out of sorts afterwards, ask yourself why you're feeling that way; try to trace the feeling back to its origins or triggers. Sometimes, just being able to understand why you're feeling the way you do can help restore your emotional equilibrium. So give yourself a brief interview and see if you can overcome the feeling by processing it. If it still bothers you, then ask yourself what you can do to help dissipate it. If you're feeling tense or angry, use relaxation techniques like deep breathing, stretching, or listening to calming music to help yourself chill. If you're feeling tired or sluggish, take an invigorating shower or have a healthy snack to help energize you. If you're feeling stressed out or overwhelmed by what's on your "To Do" list, practice positive self-talk and focus your energy on taking one step at a time, concentrating on what you're doing right now and what you can control in the present moment. (Note to self: the rest can wait.)

Appreciate your successes. Many people charge from one workout to another or one fitness goal to the next, without taking time to acknowledge, let alone appreciate, their success. That's a mistake for various reasons. For one thing, you miss the chance to take pride in what you're accomplishing and use it to build your belief in your own ability to succeed. For another, you'll gloss over a prime opportunity to use what you've just accomplished to fuel your next feat or propel your progress. "Numerous studies have shown that experiencing success in the performance of a given task enhances subsequent performance in the same task by increasing self-efficacy, or perceived competence," as endurance guru/coach Matt Fitzgerald notes in his book *How Bad Do You Want It?* In other words, believing in yourself can lead to future achievements so pause long enough to give yourself a mental fist bump or pat on the back and enjoy your success. Doing so will set you up for a positive repeat performance.

Go for a change of venue. While consistency is important, sometimes a change of scenery can breathe some fresh air or new life into your workouts and/or your eating plan. So if you usually exercise in the gym, consider taking your workouts outside now and then. Or infuse your usual workout with a dose of novelty by doing your strength-training sequence in a different order or by exercising with a friend or group of people instead of going solo. One of the best ways to ward off exercise monotony or burnout is to include variety in your workouts so don't be afraid to try new activities (Spinning, rock climbing, or kickboxing, anyone?). Similarly, you can liven up your meals simply by taking them outside, whether it's on a picnic or to the patio or deck, or by cooking with friends. Finding ways to keep your newly healthy lifestyle habits feeling fresh will help you stay on the right course.

ARMED WITH THE IDEAS PRESENTED IN THIS CHAPTER, YOU CAN FILL YOUR fitness toolkit with proven strategies that can help you crank up your mental strength while you're making dietary and workout changes that suit your body. By amping up your mental fortitude, you'll fuel your physical efforts and vice versa, creating a powerful mind-body synergy that will help you thrive. *Count on that! Use it! And fuel that dynamic interaction!* Trust the training you're doing and the process that's already pushing you out of your previous comfort zone, broadening it, and expanding your vision for yourself. Whether you realize it or not, you've sparked a positive chain reaction: taking the steps recommended in this book will help you feel fitter, stronger, and more capable and confident both physically and mentally; these effects will create a two-way feedback loop that will continue to make you feel and function better and better, both inside and out. *You've got this!*

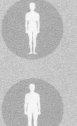

MINDFUL SHORTCUTS AND CONTINGENCY PLANS

SOMETIMES LIFE THROWS YOU CURVEBALLS OR FINDS OTHER WAYS to interfere with your schedule and best intentions. Common hiccups can include deadline crunches, vacations, business trips, out-of-town visitors, celebrations, and other circumstances that challenge your habits to stay, well, habitual. In those instances, you might stray from your diet and exercise program and end up putting yourself on a major guilt trip or taking your lapse as license to give up on your goal entirely. Both of these moves are completely unnecessary, not to mention counterproductive. The truth is, a lapse doesn't need to throw a wrench in your plans, nor does it need to lead to a complete collapse.

The key is to arm yourself with smart strategies for staying on course and pinch-hitting tactics to help you continue to reset your body chemistry and strive toward the physiological changes you want to achieve. These are not a substitute for the main approach. What I'm talking about here is more of a Plan B or contingency arrangement—a modified version of the real deal—that allows you to keep making progress when you're in a time crunch or dealing with stress overload, rather than kicking your entire program to the curb.

The reality is, you don't have to follow your personal body type plan perfectly every single day or every single week; you can take mindful detours and still grab ahold of the prize you're seeking. You can ease up by venturing into a 90/10 ratio, where you stick with the program 90 percent of the time and relax your discipline 10 percent; or, you can make it an 80/20 rule. Before they started working with me, many of my clients were working out *too* hard, restricting their food intake *too* severely, or not getting enough rest and sleep. As a result, their body chemistry was thrown off-balance—and so were their mood and energy level.

Learning *how* and *when* to let go is a critical part of my approach because you need a program that you can follow on a continuous basis. It's fine to go through strict phases for four to six weeks, but to stick with the body-type plan that's best for you or maintain your hard-won results, you need to ease up now and then so you won't burn out. With the backup plans and short-term shortcuts that follow, you'll be able to make smart choices that will, at the very least, keep your body from entering panic or rebellion mode. You will be able to maintain your latest weight and strength level while staying healthy. Even if you're not necessarily making progress in a continuous fashion, this Plan B approach will help you avoid falling off your program or taking steps backward. But the key is not to lose sight of your long-term goals in order to get back to your basic approach ASAP.

One of my clients, a mesomorph, was working on a TV show in South America and we had to adapt his diet to the food that's available in Brazil. He took photos of the markets he had access to, and we customized a meal plan based on what was there—lots of fresh fruits and veggies, and good-quality rice, beans, and meat. As for a workout venue, there was an outdoor community gym that had only free weights (no machines), so he did squats, deadlifts, bench presses, and shoulder presses with some adapted accessory moves that allowed him to do three to five exercises per muscle group; he would go on hikes to get his cardio workouts. After being away for three months, he actually came back leaner and stronger. He is proof positive that it's possible to stray from the prescribed path and still thrive!

Whenever you need some flexibility in your life, you can default to the Plan B approach that follows, up to two days a week (on a regular basis) or if you're really in a pinch for up to two weeks at a time without backsliding dramatically. Think of this as *the least you can do* to maintain or continue the progress you've been making. The tricks and hacks included here are specifically designed to maintain stable hormone and energy levels, which ultimately are what control your mood, hunger, metabolism, and other bodily sensations and functions.

On the dietary front, your best bet is to stick with 1,500 to 2,500 calories per day, depending on your age, gender, activity level, and other factors (a quick review of the "Metabolism Math" section in Chapter Three can guide you). It's also wise to have a medium carb, medium fat, and high protein intake—your diet should consist of roughly 30 to 35 percent of each macronutrient—to balance your hormones and optimize lean muscle growth and maintenance and fat loss. To make it simple, you can adopt the eating style that's been dubbed IIFYM (short for *If It Fits Your Macros*), where the idea is that as long as you eat a set amount of fat, carbs, and protein every day, your meals can consist of whatever you'd like (you can read more about it in Chapter Five).

Unless you're an ectomorph, however, try to limit your carbs to the first half of the day and/or pre- and post-workout when you'll be in peak carb-burning mode. Most people naturally consume 50 percent (or more) of their daily calories as carbs, so bringing more protein and fat into your meals will increase satiety and stabilize your insulin and blood sugar levels. Another advantage to this approach is that it's fairly easy to "eyeball" creating a plate that's made up of one-third of each macronutrient—but remember that fat contains 9 calories per gram, compared to 4 calories per gram for protein and carbs, so the proportion of fat in a meal will look significantly smaller. Because cooking oils and nut butters are so dense in calories, I strongly urge you to measure your servings of these items; otherwise, they could easily hijack your calorie intake.

Aim to include three meals and two snacks per day, to keep your calorie intake fairly consistent throughout the day. Here's what this might look like for someone who's consuming 1,500 calories per day:

MEALS	CARBS	PROTEIN	FAT	CALORIES
½ cup cooked oatmeal with 1 cup berries; 2 cooked eggs on the side	40 g	18 g	12 g	340
Protein shake (made with 1 scoop high-quality protein powder and water)	3 g	25 g	1 g	130
4 ounces cooked chicken breast, ½ sweet potato, tossed salad with 1 tablespoon extra-virgin olive oil vinaigrette	30 g	30 g	15 g	370
4 ounces broiled fish, spinach/kale salad, ½ cup cooked brown rice	30 g	35 g	15 g	450
High-protein, low-sugar energy bar (like Quest or thinkThin)	4 g net carbs	20 g	8 g	200

Note: You also can have as many veggies as you want (except bell peppers, carrots, corn, and root vegetables because they rapidly raise blood sugar) and one to two small apples and 1 to 2 cups of blueberries and/or raspberries per day.

If you don't like the look of this menu, don't sweat it. You can switch out any of those foods with the replacements in the chart that follows, as long as you swap carb for carb, protein for protein, and fat for fat and keep the serving size consistent. If the chart looks familiar, well, that's because it is—it's the same one you saw on the specific body-type plans (hey, I'm very big on consistency for the simple reason that it brings results). The difference with the Plan B approach is that you'll stick with this approach 80 to 90 percent of the time and can give yourself a free pass for 10 to 20 percent of your eating occasions.

CARBS	PROTEINS	FATS
½ sweet potato	4 ounces chicken or turkey	1 ounce nuts (small handful)
1 slice Ezekiel bread	2 eggs	1 ounce seeds (pumpkin, chia, sprouted)
½ cup cooked oats	4 ounces fish	2 eggs
½ cup cooked brown rice	1 cup broccoli, lentils, organic tofu/tempeh, or black beans	1 tablespoon coconut oil
½ cup cooked quinoa	1 scoop protein powder	1 tablespoon olive oil

People often ask me whether they can have a cocktail or two while they're working to transform their body—and the answer is, yes. You *can* work alcoholic beverages into your diet in moderation, but first consider how important it is to you to have them because the extra calories do add up and alcohol can affect your hormones temporarily. I'm not the lifestyle police, nor am I a teetotaler; I drink a glass of red wine about twice a week, and at events I'll have a cocktail or two maybe once a month. But I make it a policy to never have more than two drinks, and I strongly suggest you adopt this guideline, too. (Also, drink extra water for the sake of hydration.) Taking this approach allows you to lead a healthy, happy life—without throwing your body out of balance or disturbing your sleep.

WHAT YOU NEED TO KNOW ABOUT POPULAR SHORTCUTS

When life gets especially hectic or you feel out of control of your eating habits, in particular, you might be tempted to glom onto a fad diet. Don't do it! Many of them are based on shaky science at best or cut out so many food groups and nutrients that they're downright unhealthy. But a couple of diets du jour are worth considering—for some body types.

Intermittent fasting (IMF) is a dietary approach that's all the rage these days, and for good reason: it can work well. Giving your body "fasting periods" where it doesn't have to digest and process foods lets it dedicate internal energy and other resources to repairing your body, strengthening your immune system, and burning body fat for fuel. Another perk: people tend to eat fewer calories overall when they're doing intermittent fasting since they have fewer hours in a day in which they are permitted to eat. There are many different intermittent fasting methods. Some people eat their usual meals 5 or 6 days a week and completely fast or consume only 500 calories on the other 1 or 2 days. The more common method is to have fasting windows or periods, such as 12, 14, or 16 hours without food, accompanied by "eating-window" counterparts of 12, 10, or 8 hours, respectively. Some people narrow it down to only a 6-hour period in which they can eat.

With IMF, the basic tenets are that you consume the calories that your body needs—and I would urge you to divide them up according to the relative macronutrient proportions that are optimal for your body type—and avoid consuming any calories during the fasting periods. That means only water, seltzer, unsweetened tea, and black coffee while fasting. Doing this for 6 to 8 weeks can yield great results—and jibes with a TYPE-friendly scenario. But I use it almost exclusively with endomorphs, mesomorphs, and their hybrids. Ectomorphs and IMF can be a problematic pair because it can lead to very low energy, and, worse, it can cause them to burn too much muscle. It's not worth the risk, IMO.

Alternatively, endomorphs can follow a ketogenic diet, which is a very low-carb, high-fat regimen, for bursts of four to six weeks at a time. After a few days or a week of following this approach, your body goes into a state called ketosis because it doesn't have enough glucose (from carbs) for your cells to use for energy; instead, it burns dietary and body fat for energy and produces chemicals called ketones as a by-product. A typical keto diet is 5 to 10 percent carbs, 15 to 30 percent protein, and 60 to 75 percent fat.

The hardest part is actually getting into a state of ketosis, which requires subsisting on essentially no carbs except what comes from greens and selected vegetables, nuts, and seeds. Besides taking a toll on your enjoyment of food, this approach is not necessarily healthy for extended periods because many carbs really are good for you! But the keto diet can lead to weight loss if it's done correctly. On the other hand, if your meals are really low in carbs but not quite low enough to shift you into a state of ketosis, you may feel lethargic, irritable, or *hangry*, have a hard time sleeping, and struggle to perform well in the gym (as well as the rest of your life)—and you may not even lose weight. That said, with endomorphs who are on a time-crunched weight-loss schedule, sometimes I'll have them jump-start their progress with a six-week ketogenic phase, followed by a more sustainable approach (as described in Chapter Six).

TAKING IT ON THE ROAD

With the world becoming increasingly globalized, it's essential for many people to learn travel hacks that will help them eat well and exercise smartly, wherever they are. For example, TV commentator/host and best-selling author Van Jones splits his time between New York, DC, LA, and traveling farther afield. Typically, he is gone for one to two weeks at a time, back for three to five weeks, and so on. When he's in town, we train together three or four times per week; for the times when he's away, we have developed a road map for eating on the road and workouts that he can customize for whatever gym or hotel gym he has access to. Even after he has been traveling for a month, Van comes back looking as if he never left and is able to train as intensely as he could before he left—and that's because he's very meticulous about his health habits. Sometimes he can only work in two or three 20-minute workouts per week when he's on the road, but between that and eating well enough to keep his energy high and fat off his body, it's enough to maintain his muscle strength and definition.

Here's the advice I always give clients about making smart choices when dining out: ideally, go for a meal with a lean source of protein, lots of veggies, and healthy carbs (such as brown rice) *or* healthy fats (such as nuts)—but not both. Fish, meats, or chicken should be grilled, baked, or broiled; try to avoid marinades that are high in fat and sugar (a dry rub or light balsamic glaze is fine). Remember, the words *breaded, pan-fried, sautéed*, and *fried* = more fat. If you're not sure how an item is prepared or whether fat is added to the dish, ask your server. Choose dishes with blanched, grilled, baked, or steamed veggies, either lightly salted or seasoned with delicious spices.

While salads typically carry a health halo, when you're dining out, they can have more calories than a burger and fries. This is especially true if the salad is drowning in dressing (that's loaded with oil and sugar) or contains fried croutons, bacon, or lots of cheese. It's smart to ask for a light vinaigrette, lemon juice and olive oil, or dressing on the side.

If it's late at night and you're really hungry, opt for extra protein and veggies and fewer carbs, or include a healthy fat if one is available. If you want a "treat meal," have one, enjoy it, and plan to be back on track the next day. Desserts and fried foods are like kryptonite for healthy bodies: once in a while, it's fine to splurge, but not regularly. The unhealthy combo of bad fats and sugar (think: ice cream sundaes, cakes, onion rings, funnel cakes—you get the idea!) will spike your insulin and lead to blood sugar, cortisol, and hunger-hormone pandemonium, leaving you in a sluggish, brain-fogged, inflammation-promoting state. *No bueno!* You'd be much better off going with a healthy protein-fat combo (such as a high-quality turkey or beef jerky and pumpkin seeds, for snacks; or a dark meat poultry or fatty steak with veggies, for meals) or a protein-carb choice (a turkey and mustard tortilla wrap for a snack; grilled chicken and a baked sweet potato, for a meal).

· · · · · · · · · · · · · · · THE SCOOP ON SUPPLEMENTS · · · · · · · · · · · · · · ·

PEOPLE OFTEN ASK me whether taking supplements will help them reach their body-transformation goals faster or more healthfully. After doing extensive research on the subject, my opinion is that the vast majority of dietary supplements are next to useless—basically, they produce expensive pee (since many of them are excreted in your urine—sorry, if that's TMI). Plus, low-quality vitamins and minerals have low bioavailability and compete to be absorbed, which means that after they duke it out in your liver, little is left to enter your bloodstream. Meanwhile, many weight-loss-promoting and appetite-stimulating supplements are unsafe, and many body-building supplements are loaded with too much caffeine.

That said, there are a few supplements that can be helpful for some people or when you need a temporary boost when you're too harried or hurried to make a solid effort to eat well. At best, these can be little helpers, but they can't make up for a lousy diet. Here are the ones I like:

- Omega-3 fatty acids: Personally, I prefer the cold-pressed fish oil that should be kept in the fridge. If you don't like the taste, get the capsules. Omega 3's help with cognitive function and they're great for reducing inflammation in people of all body types (but especially ectomorphs who may struggle with ultra-sensitive adrenal glands).

- Zinc and magnesium: You can take supplements of these mighty minerals separately or with a product called ZMA, which contains zinc, magnesium, and vitamin B_6. For people who are doing heavy-duty strength training, this helps replenish depleted mineral stores, which can in turn help improve your sleep, optimize your hormone balance, and enhance your mood and cognitive function; in particular, mesomorphs who have a higher muscle content can benefit from taking these.

- Apple cider vinegar (ACV): Some research suggests that drinking a small amount (as in 1 tablespoon) of apple cider vinegar diluted in a cup of water can lower blood sugar levels after meals and improve insulin sensitivity. While this is beneficial for any body type, it's especially useful for endomorphs who often struggle with insulin and blood sugar regulation.

- Specific vitamins and minerals: Many people, especially vegans, aren't getting enough vitamin B_6, B_9, and B_{12}; vitamin D; or choline from their diets. Depending on which nutrient(s) you may be short on, it would be better to take these supplements selectively and separately than to go with a low-grade multivitamin-mineral supplement; you could, however, invest in a good-quality B-complex supplement.

- Spirulina and chlorella: These are different forms of algae and they're packed with vitamins, minerals, amino acids, protein, and other nutrients. Personally, I add these to my protein shakes as a health-boosting superfood.

- Branched chain amino acids: A staple in the bodybuilding world, I use and recommend BCAA supplements to people who want to build and maintain swole (a.k.a. jacked) muscles while cutting calories. You can take these supplements during workouts and/or when you're feeling a little hungry but you have already met your food intake for the day. BCAA can help take off the hunger edge while also preserving muscle, thus encouraging your body to burn fat as fuel instead of muscle.

• • •

YOUR BASIC TRAINING

When your schedule is cramped or you can't get to the gym on the regular, remember that doing something physical is always better than doing nothing. Ideally, when time is short, we're looking for the biggest "bang for your buck," a workout that promotes fat burning and muscle stimulation in an efficient manner. One of the best approaches you can take involves a combination of cardio (such as jogging or walking briskly for 30 minutes three times per week or 15 minutes of an HIIT circuit or Tabata workout, three times per week), along with body-weight-based strength-training moves two or three days per week. This blended workout approach will optimize fat loss and boost muscle strength. Best of all, it can be done anywhere (no gym required!) because all you need is your body.

For the HIIT circuit, you'll want to perform each of the following moves consecutively, rest for 30 seconds, then repeat the circuit as many times as you can in 15 minutes:

10 Burpees (without Push-Ups)
10 Squats
30 seconds of Jumping Jacks
10 Push-Ups
10 Supermans
10 V-Ups

TABATA TRAINING

For a super-efficient cardio workout that's a variation on the HIIT theme, try a Tabata workout (developed by Japanese scientist Izumi Tabata, Ph.D., at the National Institute of Fitness and Sports in Tokyo). It has a 2:1 work-to-rest ratio that is challenging to both your aerobic and anaerobic energy levels, resulting in improved cardiovascular fitness. You can do Tabata training on your favorite cardio machine (an indoor cycle, treadmill, elliptical, or rowing machine) or while running or walking outside in just 14 minutes! Cardio machines have timers on them that you can use to monitor your intervals; if you're doing Tabata or HIIT outside, use a stopwatch or a timer app on your phone.

Here's how:

5-minute warm-up, working at 40 percent of your maximum effort

20 seconds, 100 percent maximum effort

10 seconds rest

20 seconds, 100 percent maximum effort

10 seconds rest

20 seconds, 100 percent maximum effort

10 seconds rest

20 seconds, 100 percent maximum effort

10 seconds rest

20 seconds, 100 percent maximum effort

10 seconds rest

20 seconds, 100 percent maximum effort

10 seconds rest

20 seconds, 100 percent maximum effort

10 seconds rest

20 seconds, 100 percent maximum effort

10 seconds rest

5-minute cool-down

For strength training when you're off your usual workout schedule, either at home or when you're traveling, I like a very simple body-weight routine because body-weight exercises are great for building strength, flexibility, and body awareness. With the routines that follow, you should have a break day between workouts 1 and 2 (don't do them on consecutive days, in other words); or, if time allows, do the HIIT circuit or Tabata cardio routine or a steady 30-minute cardio stint instead on your break day. These workouts will get your heart racing, your muscles pumping, and your body's fat-burning furnace revving high. But remember: these are your "in a pinch" workouts, not the main events that are in the specific body-type plans. One thing you may notice is that if you do these travel/in-a-pinch workouts, then go back to your usual routine when you get home, you'll be stronger than you expected because you will have been progressing without realizing it.

WORKOUT 1:

Start by doing the following moves in 10 sets or less (as in 10 sets of 10 reps). Eventually work your way up to doing them all in three or four sets (which would put your reps in the 20s or 30s). Do each exercise fully before moving on to the next one. So do 20 reps of Squats, rest for 1 minute, go back to squats, and repeat this pattern until you've done 100. Then move on to Push-Ups. If doing 100 Push-Ups is way beyond your comfort quotient or if the whole workout is taking more than 20 minutes, then drop your target to, say, 70 reps of each in that 20-minute time frame; then, as you get stronger, set your sights on 100.

100 wide-stance Squats (feet placed beyond shoulder-width apart and slightly turned out)

100 Push-Ups

100 V-Ups (You can opt for crunches if doing this many V-Ups is too hard for you.)

Stretch afterward then hit the shower.

WORKOUT 2:

Take 1-minute breaks between sets and perform each exercise fully before moving on to the next one, as you did with workout 1.

100 Triceps Dips (use a bench, chair, or anything handy)

3 sets of 30-second Bicycle Crunches, followed immediately by 20 Supermans

50 Squats (narrow stance, feet facing forward and about 6 inches apart)

25 Glute Kickbacks (with each leg)

Stretch afterward then hit the shower.

KEEPING YOUR EYES ON THE PRIZE

Hopefully, now you appreciate that sticking with the optimal diet and training approach for your body type doesn't require you to be a perfect machine. None of us is, and none of us needs to be. This is real life, and the big-picture goal is to keep it (and you) balanced, healthy, and happy. So go ahead and aim high with your body transformation goals, but stay realistic and do what makes sense for your life. Everyone gets buffeted by the stresses, strains, and ever-changing demands that come with modern living, and it's okay for you to seize the flexibility and wiggle room you need for your diet and exercise habits.

Yes, consistency is important, but so is doing whatever it takes to keep this program feeling continuously fresh and appealing. Sometimes, that means choosing Plan B for the sake of your sanity or loosening the reins of dietary restraint or exercise discipline and allowing yourself treats, time-outs, and other essential forms of self-care. Remember, you're in the driver's seat—this process really is yours—but that doesn't mean you have to put the pedal to the metal all the time or slam on the brakes. There's a healthy middle ground. Find it and embrace it. Stay flexible in your mind, spirit, and behavior, and your body will repay the favor.

NEXT-LEVEL GREATNESS

ONCE YOU'VE ACHIEVED OR MADE CONSIDERABLE PROGRESS toward your body goals, you can afford to loosen the reins on your dietary restraint, just a bit. If you're trying to lose more weight, stick with the dietary guidelines for your body type 90 percent of the time and ease up 10 percent of the time (perhaps by having a small treat a couple of times per week or giving yourself a free pass to eat whatever you'd like for a day every 10 days). Easing up is okay; easing up too much is a problem—so you'll need to hold yourself accountable. When my clients reach their goals, I continue to track their eating habits on a bi-weekly basis to make sure they're not straying off course too much (I recommend you do the same). I also ask them how they feel and what they want, to help them aim for the sweet spot where they can stay accountable and committed to their body-type breakthrough while allowing themselves to enjoy their favorite foods now and then.

By contrast, if you're trying to maintain your newly slimmed-down status, you may be able to relax your vigilance 20 percent of the time. Restricting yourself excessively is *not* the way to go because it sets you up for all-or-nothing thinking that can backfire and trigger serious lapses from the plan. But remember, too, you can't out-train a bad diet. A great workout can burn 400 to 600 calories in an hour (even more if you're going into full-blown beast mode), but that same amount of calories can be put right back into your body with 2 cups of gelato, some chips, an iced mocha with whipped cream, or even a delicious and "healthy" acai bowl (I love these but they can be 1,000 calories or more with all the fixings—a serious calorie bomb!). The point is, if you've achieved your body goal, partly through tightening up your food choices, especially if you've been focused on weight loss, if you say, "Hey, I made it!" and start regularly adding back foods and drinks that are not on the plan, you might soon find that your clothes feel a bit tight or the number on the scale has crept up. You'll find yourself backsliding, in other words.

Sure, you can relax a bit, but the goal behind this book has been to give you a balanced lifestyle that suits your body type. When you go outside it with increasing frequency, your body will slowly start to return to where it was before you made these changes. *Which is probably not what you want!*

KEEP CHALLENGING YOURSELF PHYSICALLY

Don't let your workout efforts become stagnant or stale, and don't become complacent about your physical fitness goals or your accomplishments. As you get stronger and fitter, you'll notice that the workouts you've been doing have become easier. That's a good thing as well as a bad thing. On the upside, it means that you've made major progress and that what used to be challenging for your body no longer is. The downside: this means that your muscles, lungs, and heart have adapted to the program and you are no longer getting as many cardio-boosting, strength-building, or fat-burning benefits as you did initially. This is a normal part of the overload-adaptation cycle that comes with physical training. When your current workouts consistently feel easy to you, that's a sign that you need to take them to the next level or you'll wind up stuck on an exercise plateau (reaping lackluster perks, in other words!). At that point, the key is to confuse or surprise your muscles or your heart by introducing more intense segments to your workouts, making your workouts longer or faster than they are now, adjusting the amount of weight you're using or the reps you're doing, or adding challenging new forms of exercise to your current regimen. Whatever your personal body type is, making these changes will essentially jump-start your body's fitness gains once again and help your heart, lungs, and muscles continue to thrive.

You can also tweak your body-type program in key ways to take your progress to the next level. Here's how:

Ectomorphs

Until now, you've been focusing on building muscle—and you've probably got some new definition to show for it. Congrats! The focus of your workouts was initially on doing compound movements with heavy weights to add volume to your frame, followed by isolated accessory movements to shape those long limbs and add some curves. You've been avoiding lots of cardio to avoid burning too many calories (and losing muscle) and to keep your sensitive adrenal hormones in check—it's all to the good!

Now comes the more advanced part: we're going to implement three different techniques—time under tension (which refers to how long a particular muscle is under strain during a set) to help you gain muscle faster; plyometric (a.k.a. jump training) movements to increase your speed, strength, and power; and medium-level calisthenics (using your own body weight to help you get stronger)—to help you continue to build your dream physique. Your next-level program will *look* similar, but *feel* completely different—as in, much harder (*sorry not sorry*).

For the first technique, you will continue the muscle-building ectomorph workout—but change *every* exercise to a 5-second eccentric movement (the "going down" part) and a 2-second concentric movement (the "going up" part). This technique utilizes the principle of time under tension, which essentially means the more time that your muscle is under stress, the more muscle fibers are recruited, and the more benefits you will reap in terms of muscle growth. (Note: this is not very effective for power or strength training, but this is a next-level technique specifically for muscle growth.) Don't be alarmed: with this technique, the amount of weight you lift and the number of reps you do will naturally decrease dramatically—and that's okay. Start by following the same protocol for reps and sets, but adjust them as needed: if you were using 25-pound dumbbells for three sets of 10 reps on shoulder presses, don't be surprised if that comes down to 20 pounds or even 15 pounds at first. The slowed-down exercises are much, much more difficult; they're supposed to be. Stick with this technique for a 6 to 8 week periodization phase, and you'll soar over your fitness plateau with ease.

The second and third techniques (plyometric movements and medium-level calisthenics, respectively) are different, but complementary. These are body-weight-based training methods. With plyometrics (plyo), the focus is on increasing power (think squat jumps, box jumps, ladder hops, and the like), whereas calisthenics are more flexibility- and strength-oriented (think L-sits, levers, handstands, etc.). Both techniques are extremely effective at increasing your body's strength, agility, and quickness capabilities and helping you create a tighter, faster, stronger, more defined body. *Who doesn't want that?!* You've already done some of both of these types of movements in your workouts or HIIT trainings, but now you're going to add some structure and difficulty to the picture.

Plyometrics workouts: Box jumps, squat jumps, push-ups with an explosive push off the floor (clap if you can), burpees with knee tuck (bringing your knees to your chest when you jump up), lunge jumps. Treat this like a shorter HIIT workout.

Calisthenics: Pistol squats, L-sits, handstands (practice against a wall), triceps triangle push-ups, hand walk-outs. Work up to doing three sets of 10 reps on the movements, and 30-second holds on the L-sit and handstand. If you can do handstands, try doing handstand push-ups (also on the wall) until you have strong enough balance to try them without the wall.

You can sprinkle these workouts in anywhere you'd like with your existing workout days, or do them before or after a cardio session of your choice. The beauty of these next-level routines is that you can mix and match them, doing some or all three. The time under tension regimen is designed to maximize muscle, so if that's no longer the goal you can skip it. Plyometrics and calisthenics are notoriously hard for long-limbed ectomorphs so they're a great way to push your limits—or you can combine calisthenics and plyo for a 20- to 30-minute workout one or two days per week. Remember, these workouts aren't the foundation of your exercise regimen, so use them when you have extra time or energy but not at the expense of the primary stuff. Try them a couple times per week to build up your technique and endurance. I promise, you will build crazy core strength with these, more than if you did sit-ups all day long. Between doing slow, meticulous reps with the time under tension technique on your weight days and powerful, strong movements when you mix in plyometrics or calisthenics, you'll find you are pushing yourself to new heights without even realizing it.

One of my clients, actor Alan Ruck (from HBO's *Succession* and the movie *Ferris Bueller's Day Off*), has reached the north side of 60, and he can do 10 full pull-ups. After hitting the gym hard with me for a year, he started traveling for work for months at a time; while he was away, we focused on having him do a full body-weight plyo/calisthenics program instead of going to the gym, and he was able to get stronger than ever with just 30 minutes of a plyo-calisthenics combo three times per week, plus daily brisk walks. Alan is a pure ectomorph who was threatening to tip over the edge into ecto-endomorph territory, and he totally transformed his body and strength; then, he maintained his newly muscular body with these advanced techniques.

Mesomorphs

In some ways, it's hard to imagine mesomorphs needing to up their game. After all, they've already got muscles, they burn fat efficiently, and they reap progress quickly from their workouts—but even they are not immune to plateaus. To take progress to the next level with mesomorphs, I usually go one of two ways—by doubling down on the cardio or the weights route. In terms of volume, I'll add about 20 percent more distance or duration with the cardio, but I try to really push the limits with intensity (by giving maximum effort on hill sprints, body-weight HIIT or Tabata workouts, or cardio machines and ending each cardio session with a few minutes of a push-to-failure level of intensity). Since mesomorphs have muscle-sparing bodies, there's less of a concern about over-training and depleting muscle glycogen reserves. If a mesomorph wants to get *really* toned, with washboard abs, we'll go through a "conditioning phase," in which they'll do morning cardio workouts (under fasting conditions; as in—no breakfast!) at a brisk uphill pace (such as speed 4 and incline 4 on a treadmill) for 30 to 45 minutes. While the jury is still out on whether exercising on an empty stomach makes you burn more body fat, since mesomorphs have more muscle, they will burn more body fat in a fasted state than if they were to exercise after eating. It allows your body to get into stubborn fat stores more quickly than when you have food or glycogen to burn first. Plus, after you've worked out in a fasted state, the food (protein/carbs) you consume post-workout is directly used to replenish your glycogen stores and your muscle.

Diet wise, I'll encourage my mesomorph clients to implement a 16-hour fast, followed by an 8-hour eating window (with the same recommended macronutrients and calories during the eating phase). Their weight training will continue as usual—sticking with whatever plan they were doing, unless they really need to vary it because they're bored or they have specific new goals. This consistent approach really tightens up the body, allowing toned muscle to shine as the fat melts off.

If getting to the next level of muscle is the goal because you want to look jacked for a show, an event, or a competition, then we will increase the volume of sets and reps per muscle group and further isolate which body parts are addressed on which days. If calorie intake, macronutrient levels, and sufficient rest are all in check, a mesomorph can lift weights up to 5 days a week, which means we are adding both an entire day of exercise and more total volume. This is in line with the principle of progressive overload (to refresh your memory, go back to Chapter Three, if you need to). For serious muscle growth, I would typically split a mesomorph 5-day plan into something like this (though, the spacing or timing may change based on day 5 choices):

Day 1: Chest and Core. Try adding alternating one-arm/one-leg Push-Ups and Planks using a ball.

Day 2: Back/Forearms/Calves. Do 6 sets of 15 to 20 reps on calf raises, wrist curls, and reverse flies.

Day 3: Legs (Hamstring, Quads, Glutes) and Abs. Try adding Pistol Squats and Single-Leg Romanian Deadlifts to tone the smaller, stabilizing muscles.

Day 4: Arms (Shoulders, Biceps, Triceps). Address the muscle you want to get the most results with first on this day, then proceed in a prioritized fashion. Shoot for 15 sets of moves per muscle, alternating between muscle groups to keep your arms pumped; focus less on the weight amount here. For example, you might do back-to-back sets of Standing

Dumbbell Biceps Curls, Lateral Raises, and Triceps Kickbacks, for 10 to 15 reps of each; after completing the series of three moves, take a 45-second break then repeat the series two more times.

Day 5: Double-up Day. Pick the two body parts you want to maximize your results on and do the same exercises as on the other days but mixing and matching the moves so they address your goals. For example, if you want to develop toned abs and more leg definition, you could pair up Planks and Pistol Squats.

Whether your next goal is to become extra toned or extra muscled, the key for a mesomorph is to increase the total volume of your workouts by upping the frequency. But remember to listen to your body because rest, recovery, and the right calories are essential for fueling these workouts. If you find that you're not performing well, check out these factors first before you decide this approach is just too hard. Then, readjust your habits and reevaluate the workout as necessary. By this point, you likely have a much better handle on what your body can do and what it needs, which means you can adjust your current mesomorph workout on your own. Give it a shot; you can always fine-tune your approach along the way.

Endomorphs

While it's especially true at the beginning, dietary changes will continue to rule the day for endomorphs who want to slim down and shape up. There's just no getting around that. That means you can continue to follow the endomorph plan (from Chapter Six) if it's working for you; or, if you need an extra boost, I would highly recommend intermittent fasting for six to eight weeks, whether you want to lose fat or gain muscle. Start with a 14-hour fast, followed by a 10-hour window for eating, and try to stick to the same schedule daily to optimally manage your satiety and hunger levels. Maybe you'd fast from 7 p.m. until 9 a.m. then divvy up your meals and snacks between 9 a.m.

and 7 p.m. While doing this, you'll want to make sure you continue following the macronutrient guidelines for endomorphs. Remember, this is an advanced technique that you could try assuming you've already trained and eaten properly for your body type the basic way. If that's not the case, you may feel tired, foggy, and aggravated trying to do intermittent fasting before you have stabilized your leptin, ghrelin, and insulin levels through months of healthy living. Don't try to run before you can walk! (It's not safe.)

From a training standpoint, you'll want to keep your low-intensity cardio workouts going as often as possible, and do weight-training workouts three or four times per week. The most effective advanced technique for boosting an endomorph to the next fitness level is really focusing on bringing up the level and frequency of HIIT workouts that are being performed: whether it's a high-intensity Spin class, a Tabata workout, or hill sprints (my favorite), getting your HIIT sessions up to three or even four times a week is a great way to keep burning body fat for fuel and staying mentally and physically on top of your game.

If you want to get super advanced and do Olympic and powerlifting style movements like cleans, clean and jerks, and snatches (you may have seen these on YouTube, at CrossFit gyms, or in Olympic competitions), I recommend working with a coach or trainer who can teach you the proper form for these movements. Endomorphs have great power and muscle fibers that are well tuned for these movements, but there are precise techniques for each of these. If you don't do them correctly, you could get injured (hence the need for supervision by a pro). But if you do them the right way, your muscles will pulse and tighten, and you'll continue to chisel out your physique—and look downright badass!

NEXT-LEVEL MOTIVATION

As you make additional progress with your body-type plan, continue to seek out physical activities that make you feel vibrant and strong or that challenge your body or mind in all the right ways. (Think of them as physical fun.) Continue to find the fire inside you and strive to achieve new personal bests, to push your limits and expand your comfort zone in the fitness arena and in the rest of your life, so that you can create the absolute best version of yourself. This way you can feel happy and proud of yourself, which brings its own brand of positive reinforcement. Remember, you're the one who's holding the keys and sitting in the driver's seat with your hands on the steering wheel. You've got the strength, power, and know-how in your body and mind to guide you to the next destination, whatever or wherever it might be. So, set your sights on your target and rely on your physical and mental strength and prowess to drive you to the prizes of better health, fitness, and a happier, more gratifying life. You deserve nothing less!

CONCLUSION

JUST YOUR TYPE IS REALLY ABOUT WORKING SMARTER, NOT necessarily harder, and taking full possession of your body as you strive to help it become the best version of itself possible. Once you're happy with your body-fat level and your new eating habits, you can modify the program somewhat and fine-tune it so that it works optimally for you. After all, I want you to own this program and view it as your new normal, not some fad regimen that gets ditched or fades away. So, don't be afraid to switch up the order of your strength-training moves, lift more weight with fewer reps (or vice versa), or choose different cardio workouts to challenge yourself in new ways while staying true to the spirit of the body-type principles that are right for you. Small changes like these will help you reignite muscle growth and keep your workouts feeling fresh. With this kind of flexibility, it won't feel like you're doing the same workout day after day, which can start to feel monotonous. Keep giving yourself choices.

To keep things feeling fresh, it also can help to find a workout buddy who's on a similar fitness level or similarly motivated. Even if you have different body types, you can work out together, coach each other, and cheer each other on. If you're new to a particular gym, you might want to look for a fitness mentor there, someone you can ask for helpful tips or strategies when your own motivation starts to wane. You don't have to do this alone!

It also helps to set your sights on new goals—perhaps an anniversary goal six months or a year into your body-type-enhancing program. Now that you've started to develop greater body confidence, consider what you'd like to do with it. Maybe it's trying something new (like rock climbing, boxing, hip-hop dancing, aerial yoga, or a boot-camp-style workout) that you didn't have the guts to do in the past. Or maybe you want to compete in a half-marathon or triathlon or a Tough Mudder race. Perhaps you'd like to take an adventure vacation (like trekking in Nepal, glacier hiking in Iceland, cycling through Tuscany, or sailing in the Greek Islands). It's your choice. There's no need to share your next-level goal with anyone if you don't want to; simply whisper it to yourself or write it down in a journal. Remind yourself of it when you need an infusion of inspiration.

Above all, try to remember that this really is about *you*; so make a concerted effort to understand what makes *your* body feel strong and comfortable and how you can challenge it smartly. Don't go rogue and just grab a move or a workout you see someone else doing in the gym without understanding the foundation that particular person has built for doing it and why it's appropriate for him or her. I see this mistake being played out again and again at the gym—and it's problematic because your fitness foundation and needs may be quite different, which means that ripping off someone else's regimen could cause you to hurt yourself, burn out, or lead to muscle imbalances. Also, don't become a diet or workout surfer: it's fine to mix things up now and then (just like you do with your wardrobe on casual Fridays), but most of the time you should be sticking with the same good-for-you habits—the ones your body responds to best. Your body needs and thrives on consistency—it's really that simple.

In my experience, consistency with training and structure around meals are two of the most important ingredients for achieving body transformation. (The others are focus, determination, perseverance, and enthusiasm.) Without these supporting players, it will be much harder for you to reach your fitness goals. Even once you've achieved your strongest, fittest body, don't throw away those key ingredients—hold onto them!—so you can maintain your newly impressive physique. People who prioritize their health do the best at transforming their bodies. That means you need to plan for health-related activities, just like you would an important business meeting. Schedule it on your calendar, and make it a sacred appointment with yourself. Continue to set new objectives for yourself, whether it's to run faster, climb higher, or hoist more weight. And continue to ask yourself why these new goals matter to you so that you can infuse them with intrinsic motivation and meaning (or purpose). Also, be sure to treat your body right by getting enough sleep and taking time for relaxation and stress-management measures to help your body and mind restore and rejuvenate themselves.

One of the welcome side effects of a body-type approach to improving your health and fitness level is that you'll stop judging your body and start embracing it, which has positive consequences in terms of how you treat it, talk about it, and think about it. After a workout or a particularly difficult set, get in the habit of giving yourself a head nod in the mirror, a visual high-five that signals approval. When you continuously notice fairly dramatic results from your training, the conversation in your head will change and you'll come to feel differently about your body. Maybe you've even begun to discover new facets of what your body can do and found ways to maximize your physique's strength and power in everyday life. That's as it should be, because this is the only body you're ever going to have so it's in your best interest to treat it and think about it positively and to show it some love on a daily basis.

Ultimately, think of this program as an investment in fulfilling your fitness potential and extending the quality of your life well into the future. By challenging your body and fueling it properly, you really can create a positive ripple effect of feel-good perks. In the process of working to strengthen your body and your mind, you have embarked on a journey of self-discovery, one that has undoubtedly started to broaden the way you view yourself, not just in the mirror but in your mind's eye as well. As you gain greater self-confidence and a more defined vision of yourself, you'll develop a stronger sense of ownership in your body, and that will help you feel empowered to make better choices for yourself.

Take pride in the new version of yourself that you're becoming, and you'll move through the world with greater ease and your comfort zone will broaden in nearly every aspect of your life. Besides enhancing your health and energy, you'll ramp up the pleasure you get from looking, feeling, and functioning at your absolute best. That's just about the greatest gift you could give yourself because it doesn't stop giving. *Not. Ever.*

A NOTE FROM THE AUTHOR

I HOPE YOU'VE ENJOYED *JUST YOUR TYPE*, WHICH IS BASED ON THE motivating, no-nonsense, customized approach I use to sculpt and enhance the physiques of my celebrity clients, media stars, and others. In addition to training people in Hollywood or online, I am the co-founder of Tranzend Health (www.tranzendhealth.com), a wellness supplements company, and my brother, Dave Catudal, who's also a celebrity trainer and health expert, and I have a business called Airlean (https://airlean.com/) that aims to revolutionize healthy travel.

Many of my clients travel frequently, and when they're away, some will send me pictures of their film set or hotel gym so I can design a workout that they can do there; if no equipment is available, I'll create a hotel-room workout for them. I will also help them create healthy meal plans based on the foods that are available at their location. Airlean developed from this concept. Through this venture, we have worked with Hollywood stars, European royalty, politicians, business moguls, pilots, cabin crew, doctors, lawyers, architects, and even other self-help gurus. If you travel frequently, I urge you to check it out.

If you've enjoyed the book or you want a little extra training info, feel free to let me know. I'd be happy to continue the conversation through my website (http://www.trainedbyphil.com/). You also can find new tips or motivation strategies by following me on Instagram (@TrainedByPhil). Looking forward to hearing from you!

APPENDIX A

THE EXERCISES

Y OU'VE ARRIVED: HERE'S YOUR GUIDE TO THE DIFFERENT EXER-
cises I have described throughout the book, with step-by-
step instructions for how to do them correctly. Good form is
essential—I cannot emphasize that enough, because it can mean
the difference between getting the results you want and not. So,
get familiar with the deets that follow and stay true to them!

· · · · · · · · · · GET INTO MODIFY MODE! · · · · · · · · · ·

IF YOU'RE INTIMIDATED by some of these moves or
worried that you won't be able to do certain exercises, don't be afraid to modify them.

- If you can't do full push-ups, do them from your knees.

- If you can't squat until your thighs are parallel to the ground, squat onto a box or chair or place a large exercise ball between you and a wall to assist you.

- If pull-ups are impossible for you, use a pull-down or assisted pull-up machine or use resistance bands for assistance.

- For hack squats, deadlifts, and other dumbbell, barbell, or free weight lifts, I do want you to follow my plans as written. But almost all of the free weight exercises that involve a dumbbell or barbell have machine equivalents; these may be easier for you to use initially.

The point is, whatever the exercise is, there is a way to get benefits and start off on the right foot even if you can't do it exactly as prescribed at first. So keep working at it and you'll make progress sooner than you think.

• • •

SQUATS

Stand with your feet hip-width apart, with your knees, hips, and toes facing forward, your head and shoulders up, and your abs braced. As you bend your knees, lower your hips and butt, as if you were going to sit in a chair, and raise your arms straight out in front of you to shoulder level. (Keep your weight on your heels, not your toes; your thighs should be parallel to the floor and your knees shouldn't extend past your toes.) Hold the squat for a count or two then rise back up to standing. Repeat.

WEIGHTED SQUATS

Repeat the same move as the basic squat while holding dumbbells in each hand.

BARBELL SQUATS

Place a barbell on a squat rack so that it's at the same height as your upper chest. Position your body under the barbell, with your back to the rack and your knees bent, so that the barbell is resting high up on the backs of your shoulders. Hold the bar with an overhand grip at a distance that's comfortably wider than your shoulders and slowly straighten your legs to lift the barbell from the rack. Take a step away from the rack and stand with your feet shoulder-width apart. Bend your knees and push your hips and butt back (as if you were going to sit) until your thighs are parallel to the floor. Pause for a count, then push up through your heels as you straighten your hips and knees until you are back to a standing position (with your knees slightly bent). Repeat.

FRONT (BARBELL) SQUATS

Position your body under a barbell on a squat rack, with your knees bent, so that the barbell is resting on the fronts of your shoulders. Bring your elbows up and hold the bar with an overhand grip shoulder-width apart and slowly straighten your legs to lift the barbell from the rack. Take a step away from the rack and stand with your feet shoulder-width apart, your back flat, and your abs engaged. Bend your knees and push your hips and butt back (as if you were going to sit) until your thighs are parallel to the floor. Pause. Return to the starting position. Repeat.

HACK SQUATS

Place a loaded barbell behind you on the floor, and place two 25-pound plates under your heels. Tighten your core, keep your lower back straight, and slowly squat down and grasp the barbell behind you. Use your heels to drive yourself up to a standing position while holding the barbell behind you; keep a slight bend in your knees when you get to the top. Slowly squat again, driving your hips behind you as you lower the barbell back to the floor. Repeat.

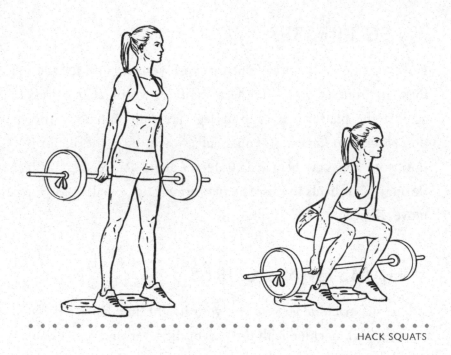

HACK SQUATS

JUMP SQUATS

Stand with your feet hip-width apart and pointing straight ahead; place your hands behind your head. Keep your weight on your heels, bend your knees, and lower your hips toward the floor, as if you were going to sit in a chair. Pause for a count or two when you reach your lowest point; then use an explosive movement to drive through your heels and push yourself up off the floor, reaching your arms overhead as you jump into the air. Land with your knees slightly bent to cushion the impact. Repeat.

LEG PRESSES

Have a seat on a leg-press machine with your legs on the platform in front of you, your feet shoulder-width apart. Press against the platform until your legs are fully extended (but don't lock your knees). As you inhale, slowly lower the platform until your knees are bent at a 90-degree angle. Pause, then push through your heels to raise the platform again, exhaling as you move. Repeat.

HAMSTRING CURLS

Adjust the machine lever to suit your height then lie face down on a leg curl machine with the pad of the lever on the backs of your lower legs (a few inches below your calves). Keep your torso flat on the bench and grab the machine's side handles. As you exhale, curl your legs up as far as you can without lifting your upper legs from the pad. At the top of the movement, pause; then slowly bring your legs back to the starting position as you inhale. Repeat.

WALKING LUNGES

Stand with your feet shoulder-width apart and hold a dumbbell in each hand. Take a big step forward with your right leg, keeping your left foot where it was, and bend your knees as you do this so that your back knee comes down toward the floor (keep your back straight as you do this). Lower yourself until your right knee is bent at a 90-degree angle. Pause. Then push down through your right heel and return to a standing position by bringing your left foot to join your right. Repeat this move with the left leg, and continue this "walking" pattern 10 paces in one direction; then turn around and do 10 paces in the other direction. (This way, each leg gets 10 lunges per set.)

SHOULDER PRESSES WITH DUMBBELLS

Stand with your feet shoulder-width apart, hold a dumbbell in each hand, and raise the dumbbells to just above shoulder level, with your palms facing forward. As you press your arms up and overhead, straighten your arms and rotate your palms inward so they're facing each other at the top. Lower the dumbbells to above shoulder level again and repeat.

LATERAL RAISES

Stand with your feet shoulder-width apart and hold a dumbbell
with an overhand grip in each hand; your arms should be hanging down at your sides with your palms facing your body. Keep
your arms straight, and as you exhale, raise your arms up and out
to the side until they are at shoulder level but not beyond. At the
top, your palms should face the floor. As you inhale, lower your
arms back down in a controlled fashion. Repeat.

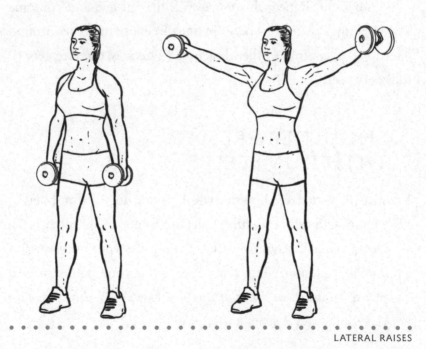

LATERAL RAISES

FRONT RAISES

Stand with your feet shoulder-width apart and hold a dumb-bell with an overhand grip in each hand; your arms should be hanging in front of your thighs with your palms facing your body. Keep your chest up and your abs engaged as you lift the dumb-bells in front of you to shoulder height. Pause, then slowly lower the dumbbells to the starting position. Repeat.

FLAT BENCH PRESS

Lie on your back on a flat bench while holding a dumbbell in each hand with an overhand grip. Start by holding the dumbbells above your shoulders, slightly wider than shoulder-width apart, with your palms facing forward. Slowly bend your elbows at a 90-degree angle (so that your upper arms are parallel to the floor). Push the weights up in an arc motion, as you straighten your arms, until the dumbbells are end-to-end above the center of your chest. Pause, then slowly lower the dumbbells by bending your elbows at a 90-degree angle again until your upper arms are slightly lower than parallel to the floor (you should feel a stretch in your chest and shoulder muscles). Repeat.

INCLINE DUMBBELL PRESSES

Set up an incline bench so that the backrest is at a 45-degree angle. Sit on the bench, holding a dumbbell in each hand with an overhand grip (palms facing away from you), with your back flat and your shoulders pushed back. Raise the dumbbells slightly above your shoulders, keeping your elbows bent at 90-degrees. Then, push the dumbbells up and away from your body, using your chest and shoulder muscles as you straighten your arms. Once the dumbbells are suspended above your chest, pause for a count, then lower the dumbbells back toward your chest as you bend your elbows. Repeat.

INCLINE CABLE FLIES

Stand between two cable stations and attach the dumbbell grip handles to the high pulleys on either side of you. Grasp the handles with each hand, using an overhand grip, and keep your arms outstretched. Bend your knees slightly and hinge forward a bit at the hips so that you are leaning forward somewhat. Keep a slight bend in your elbows (they should be a little bit behind you) and rotate your shoulders toward the center of your chest. Using a smooth motion, bring the grip handles together in front of your chest. Pause, and then slowly return to the starting position, until you feel a gentle stretch in your chest muscles. Repeat.

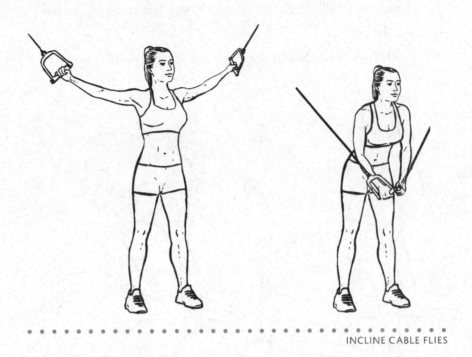

INCLINE CABLE FLIES

INCLINE DUMBBELL FLIES

Set up an incline bench to about a 30-degree angle. Lie on the bench, holding a dumbbell in each hand with an overhand grip, with your back flat and your shoulders pushed back. Bring the dumbbells above your chest and rotate your hands so that your palms are facing each other; keep your elbows slightly bent. In a smooth motion, lower both dumbbells in a wide arc out to the sides while keeping your elbows slightly bent; lower them until you feel a stretch in your chest and shoulders. Pause, and then bring the dumbbells back above your chest in a smooth, arc-like motion. Repeat.

(Note: **Dumbbell Flies** are done the same way but on a flat bench.)

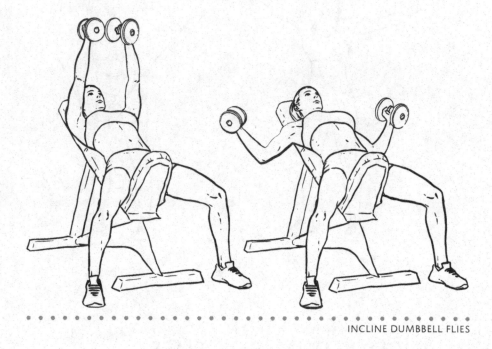

INCLINE DUMBBELL FLIES

DIPS (CHEST)

Find a pair of parallel bars (or a dip-assist machine). Start by holding the bars with each hand and pushing your body up so that your arms are fully extended. Inhale and slowly lower yourself, leaning forward with your torso about 30 degrees and your elbows flared out slightly until you feel a mild stretch in your chest. Pause, and then use your chest muscles to bring your body back to the starting position as you exhale. Repeat.

DEADLIFTS

Place a barbell in an open space on the floor and stand facing the barbell with your feet 4 to 6 inches away from the barbell and shoulder-width apart. While keeping your back straight, squat down and grasp the bar using an overhand grip (your hands should be shoulder-width apart). Keep your arms fully extended, straighten your legs, and stand up while holding the barbell; your hips and shoulders should rise together and your back should stay straight. When you get to the top of the lift, rotate your shoulders back slightly until you feel a mild stretch in them. Then lower the barbell back to the floor, using the same squatting motion that you used to lift it. Repeat.

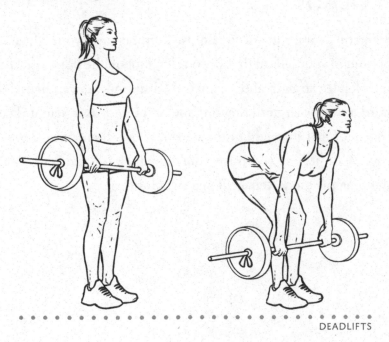

DEADLIFTS

ROMANIAN DEADLIFTS

Stand tall with your feet shoulder-width apart while holding a barbell in front of you, with your hands slightly wider than shoulder-width apart. While keeping your back flat and your core engaged, bend your knees slightly and push your hips back as your chest leans toward the floor. Keep your arms fully extended and the barbell close to your body. When you feel a contraction in the backs of your legs, slowly return to standing upright. Repeat.

SINGLE-LEG ROMANIAN DEADLIFTS

Stand on your right foot and hold a dumbbell with your left hand, in front of your left thigh. Lift your left foot off the floor and keep your left leg straight and in line with your body, as you bend forward at the waist until the dumbbell is at mid-shin height (keep your back flat throughout the move). Pause, then drive through your right heel as you push your hips forward and return to a standing position. Repeat. Then switch sides.

STIFF-LEGGED DEADLIFTS

Place a barbell on the floor and stand facing it with your feet pointed forward and shoulder-width apart and your knees slightly bent. As you exhale, bend forward at the waist while keeping your back flat and your knees slightly bent, until you feel tension in your hamstrings. Grab the barbell with an overhand grip and your hands slightly wider than shoulder-width apart. While keeping your arms fully extended, lift the barbell by extending your waist and hips in a smooth motion as you inhale, until you are standing upright again. Pause at the top, then bend forward at the waist to return the weight to the floor (or just above it). Repeat.

BENT ROWS

Stand with your feet hip-width apart and hold a dumbbell in each hand in front of you with an overhand grip; your arms should be extended and your palms should be facing each other. Tighten your core, bend your knees slightly, and hinge forward as you push your hips back so that your upper body is almost parallel to the floor. Keep your head up as you bend your elbows to a 60-degree angle and bring the dumbbells toward your chest. Pause when your upper arms are parallel to the floor, then slowly return the dumbbells to the starting position. Repeat.

UPRIGHT ROWS

Stand with your feet shoulder-width apart, with a dumbbell in each hand. Hold your arms straight down in front of you, with your palms facing your thighs. Bend your elbows and, in one smooth movement, pull both dumbbells up to just below your chin; your shoulders should stay down and back and your elbows will flare out to the side and up. When you reach the top of the movement, squeeze your biceps and forearms for a count, then lower the weights to the starting position. Repeat.

ONE-ARM DUMBBELL ROWS

Place a dumbbell on the floor on each side of a flat bench. Place your right shin on the top of one end of the bench, bend forward at the waist (until your torso is parallel to the floor), and put your right palm on the other end of the bench for support. Use your left hand to pick up the dumbbell, with the palm of your left hand facing your torso. Pull the weight straight up to the side of your chest, bending your elbow and keeping your upper arm close to your side (and your torso still). Squeeze your back muscles when you reach the full contracted position. Lower the dumbbell to the starting position. Repeat. Then switch sides.

BENT-OVER REVERSE FLIES

Stand with your feet hip-width apart, holding a dumbbell in each hand. Brace your core, bend your knees slightly, and hinge forward from the hips. Lift the dumbbells up and out to the sides to shoulder level while contracting the muscles in the back of the shoulders. Maintain a flat back and keep your elbows slightly bent throughout the movement. At the top of the movement pause, then slowly bring the dumbbells back to the starting position. Repeat.

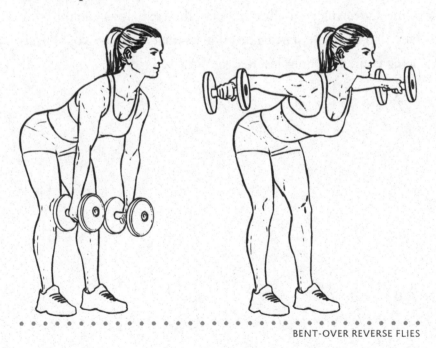

BENT-OVER REVERSE FLIES

BENCH PRESSES

Set up an incline bench in front of a weight rack so that the back-rest is at a comfortable angle and facing the weight stack. Sit on the bench, and place your back firmly against the backrest. Grasp the barbell with an overhand grip, with your hands spaced 1½ to 2 times shoulder-width apart. Lift the barbell from the rack by pushing up with your chest muscles; hold it straight above your chest with your arms fully extended. As you inhale, slowly lower the barbell until it touches your upper chest. Pause for a count while squeezing your chest muscles; then exhale as you push the barbell back to the starting position (so that it's above your chest) using your chest muscles. Repeat.

DUMBBELL PEC FLIES

Lie on your back on a flat bench, holding a dumbbell in each hand. Maintain a tight core and a flat back as you push the dumbbells straight above your chest so that the dumbbells are facing each other and touching. Keep a slight bend in your elbows, open your chest, and slowly lower the dumbbells to the sides in a wide arc out until you feel a stretch in your chest muscles and your upper arms are nearly parallel to the floor. Pause, then return to the starting position. Repeat.

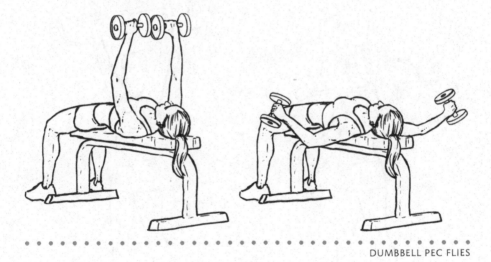

DUMBBELL PEC FLIES

MILITARY PRESSES

Place a barbell on a squat rack at shoulder height. Step under the barbell and grab it with an overhand grip, hands shoulder-width apart. Brace your core, step back while holding the barbell at shoulder height, ground your feet, and slowly push the barbell overhead (don't lock your elbows). Pause at the top, then slowly bring the barbell back to shoulder height. Repeat.

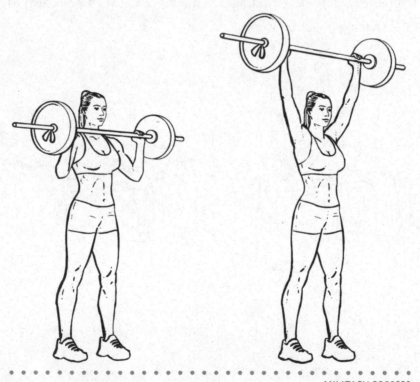

MILITARY PRESSES

BICEPS BARBELL CURLS

Stand with your feet hip-width apart, holding a barbell with an underhand grip with your hands shoulder-width apart and your arms fully extended toward the floor. Keep your elbows close to the sides of your body (your palms should be facing away from you) and curl the barbell forward and up toward your shoulders in a smooth, arc-like motion as you exhale; only your forearms should move (your upper arms should stay still). Hold the barbell for a count at the top, squeezing your biceps; then lower the barbell to the starting position as you inhale. Repeat.

HAMMER CURLS

Stand with your feet hip-width apart and your arms extended at your sides, holding a dumbbell in each hand with your palms facing in toward the sides of your body. While keeping your elbows tucked into the sides of your body, exhale and slowly curl the dumbbells up toward your shoulders by bending your elbows. (Keep your core tight and your spine straight throughout the move.) Once the dumbbells are at shoulder level, pause and squeeze your biceps, then slowly lower the dumbbells back to the starting position as you inhale. Repeat.

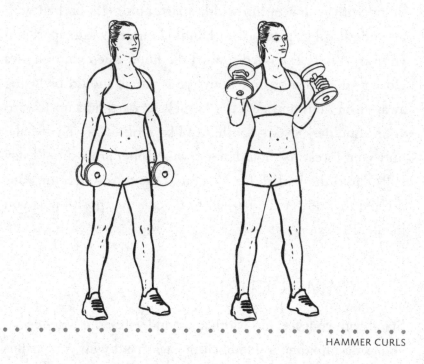

HAMMER CURLS

PREACHER CURLS

Set up a preacher curl bench, adjusting the seat so it's the right height for you. (It should be in a position so that you don't need to raise your shoulders but you don't need to lean over the support pad, either.) Place your arms on the support pad with your triceps near the top and your elbows about halfway down the pad. Hold the EZ curl bar with an underhand grip, with your hands shoulder-width apart. In a smooth, arc-like motion, curl the bar in toward your upper chest and chin. Pause for a count at the top. Then lower the bar by extending your arms fully. Repeat.

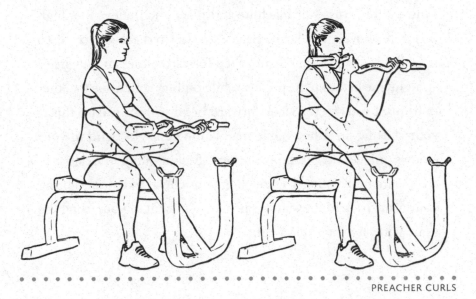

PREACHER CURLS

CABLE CURLS

Set up a cable station with a straight bar attached to the low pulley. Stand close to the apparatus, facing it, with your feet shoulder-width apart on either side of the pulley. Grasp the bar with an underhand grip, hands shoulder-width apart. While keeping your back straight and your elbows close to your sides, curl your arms upward from the elbow in a smooth, arc-like motion, continuing until the bar is at chest height. Hold this position for a count while flexing your biceps. Then lower the bar by extending your arms fully. Repeat.

CABLE CROSSOVERS

Find a cable crossover machine and place the pulleys in a high position above your head. Select the desired resistance, then hold the pulleys in each hand. Step forward along an imaginary straight line between the pulleys while pulling your arms together in front of you (keep a small forward bend in your waist): this is your starting position. While maintaining a slight bend in your elbows, inhale and extend your arms straight out to both sides in a wide arc until you feel a stretch in your chest. Exhale and bring your arms back to the starting position in front of you, using the same wide arc. Pause. Repeat.

TRICEPS PUSHDOWNS

Find a cable station with a straight bar attached to the top pulley. Stand facing the apparatus with your feet shoulder-width apart, with your knees slightly bent to stabilize your body. Hold the bar with an overhand grip, with your hands slightly less than shoulder-width apart. Pull the bar down until your forearms are parallel to the floor (around waist height) with your elbows close to your body and your wrists locked. While moving only your forearms, push the bar down toward the floor until your arms are fully extended (you should feel a stretch in your triceps). Pause for a count while squeezing your triceps, then return to the waist-high position by moving only your forearms. Pause here. Repeat.

(Note: you can do Triceps Rope Pushdowns by linking a rope attachment to the top pulley.)

SKULL CRUSHERS

Sit on a flat bench, holding a preacher curl barbell with an overhand grip. Slowly lie back until your back is flat on the bench and your feet are flat on the floor, and bring the barbell up in the air above your head. Brace your core and keep your upper arms steady (they should stay perpendicular to the floor) as you bend your elbows and slowly dip the barbell back toward your head. Pause at the bottom, then slowly push the barbell back up above your head. Repeat.

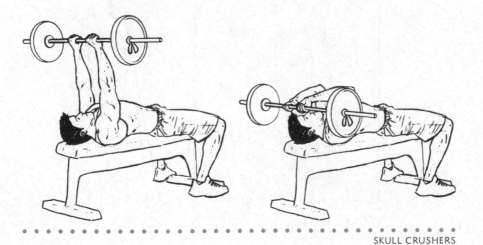

SKULL CRUSHERS

OVERHEAD TRICEPS ROPE EXTENSIONS

Connect a rope attachment to the bottom pulley of a cable station. Hold the rope with both hands, using a neutral grip, and turn your body so you're standing with your back to the apparatus, your feet hip-width apart. Extend your arms until they are directly overhead, with your hands pointing toward the ceiling. As you inhale, slowly lower the rope behind your head, keeping your elbows close to your ears and your upper arms steady (they should be in line with the sides of your body). When your triceps are fully extended, pause for a count while squeezing your triceps. As you

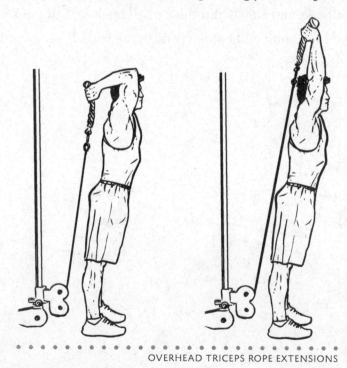

OVERHEAD TRICEPS ROPE EXTENSIONS

exhale, return to the starting position by extending your arms so your hands are pointing toward the ceiling again. Repeat.

TRICEPS DIPS

Stand between parallel bars and hold the bars with an overhand grip, keeping your elbows close to the sides of your body. Push yourself up so that your arms and shoulders are supporting your body weight. Keep your hips straight and your back flat; don't lock your elbows. Lower your body by slowly bending your elbows until they are bent at 90-degree angles and your upper arms are parallel to the floor. Pause at the low point, then push your body back up again. Repeat.

AB WHEEL ROLLOUTS

Get down on all fours on the floor and place the ab roller in front of you. Hold each end of the roller with each hand. With your abs engaged and your back flat, inhale and slowly roll the wheel forward in a straight line as far as you can without letting your torso touch the floor. Pause, then slowly roll yourself back to the starting position by exhaling and tightening your abs. Repeat.

PLANKS

Lie face down on the floor and raise yourself up onto your forearms and your toes, with your elbows positioned under your shoulders. Keep your hips raised, your back flat, and your gaze on the floor (near your hands) so that your body resembles a plank that's parallel to the floor. Squeeze your abs and glutes and hold this position for the desired time (or as long as you can). Repeat.

SIDE PLANKS

Lie on the floor on your left side with your shoulders, hips, knees, and feet in a straight line and your feet stacked on top of each other. Raise yourself up onto your left forearm so that your left shoulder is directly above your left elbow as you drive your body off the floor (you will be balancing on your forearm and the side of your lower foot); your right arm can rest along the right side of your body or you can place your right hand on your hip. Hold this side plank for the desired time, then release. Roll onto your right side and repeat the move on that side.

V-UPS

Lie on your back with your legs together and extended straight and your arms extended overhead. While keeping your back flat, use your abs to sit up while drawing your hands to touch your toes, creating a V-shape with your body. Hold this position for a count or two, then return to an extended body position without letting your heels or your shoulders touch the floor between reps. Repeat.

BICYCLE CRUNCHES

Lie on your back with your feet together, your legs extended, and your hands behind your head and your elbows wide. Lift your legs a few inches off the floor; keep your left leg straight and bend your right knee toward your upper body as you twist and touch (or almost touch) your left elbow to your right knee. Then, twist and turn so your right leg straightens and your left knee bends and touches your right elbow. Keep bringing your opposite elbow to your opposite knee in a slow, controlled fashion.

SUPERMANS

Lie face down on the floor with your legs straight and your arms extended on the floor above your head. Simultaneously raise your arms, legs, and chest a few inches off the floor and hold for 2 seconds (keep your neck in line with your body and your eyes focused on the floor)—while squeezing your glutes—then slowly return to the starting position. Repeat until you've completed the desired number of reps.

PULL-UPS

Stand under a pull-up bar, reach up, and grab the bar with an overhand grip. Your hands should be beyond shoulder-width apart. Hang from the bar with your arms straight, then while keeping your body straight, pull your body up toward the bar by pulling your elbows down toward your waist. Continue lifting yourself until your chest nearly touches the bar, and then slowly lower your body to the starting position. Repeat.

PUSH-UPS

Start at the top of a push-up, with your hands on the floor, a little more than shoulder-width apart and aligned with your chest muscles; the balls of your feet should be on the floor and your heels in the air. While engaging your abs and glutes and keeping a straight line from your head to your heels, bend your arms and lower your body toward the floor until your elbows are bent at 90-degree angles and your upper arms are parallel to the floor. Then, push yourself back up to the starting position and repeat.

LAT PULLDOWNS

Find a cable station with a straight bar attached to the top pulley. Sit on the seat facing the weights, with your feet flat on the floor and your back straight. Reach up and hold the bar with an overhand grip with your hands about 1½ to 2 times your body-width apart. Lean back slightly (but don't arch your back) and pull the bar down toward the top of your chest, using your shoulder muscles while letting your elbows arc out to the sides. When you reach the low point of the movement, pause for a second and squeeze your shoulder blades together; then slowly return to the starting position by letting the bar rise as you relax your shoulders and fully extend your arms again. Repeat.

BURPEES (A.K.A. SQUAT THRUSTS)

Stand with your feet shoulder-width apart and your hands by your sides. In one fluid motion, squat down and place your palms on the floor in front of your feet. Lean forward, placing your weight on your hands, while jumping your legs out behind you until your legs and your arms are fully extended. Your body should be in a straight line from your head to your heels, with your weight supported by your toes and the balls of your feet, as well as your hands. (You'll be in a push-up position, in other words.) Jump your feet forward so they're just behind your hands and use an explosive movement, pushing off from your heels, to propel yourself into the air, reaching your arms overhead. Return to the starting position. Repeat.

GLUTE KICKBACKS

Get down on all fours (on your hands and knees) with your back flat and your head in line with your spine. Tighten your ab muscles as you kick your right leg back and up behind you, with your foot flexed, until your right leg is in a straight line with your body.

Slowly return your leg to the starting position but don't let your right knee touch the ground. Do the desired number of reps with your right leg, then switch to your left leg. (To make this move more challenging, you can use an ankle weight or a resistance band looped around the foot being kicked back.)

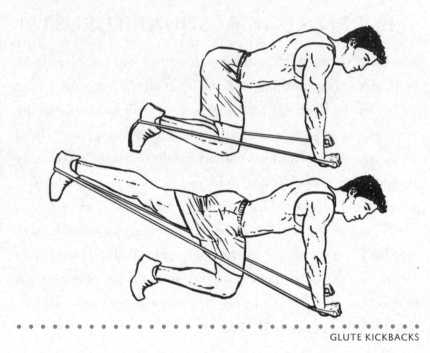

GLUTE KICKBACKS

MOUNTAIN CLIMBERS

Place your palms on the floor shoulder-width apart. Extend your legs behind you so that only your toes and the balls of the feet are touching the floor. Your body should be in a straight line with your weight on your hands and toes, with your back flat and your head in line with your spine (think plank position). Bend your right knee and hip and bring your right knee up toward your chest (your left leg should remain fully extended). With an explosive movement, switch the position of your legs so that your left knee bends and comes up toward your shoulder as your right leg jumps to an extended position behind you. Continue repeating this pattern.

TRICEPS KICKBACKS

Hold a dumbbell in each hand with your palms facing the sides of your body. While keeping your back flat and a slight bend in your knees, bend forward at the waist until your torso is almost parallel to the floor. Bend your elbows at 90-degree angles and keep your upper arms close to your torso and parallel to the floor. While keeping your upper arms steady (they should stay parallel to the floor), exhale and use your triceps to push the dumbbells straight behind you until your arms are fully extended. Pause at the top of the extension, then slowly lower the dumbbells back down until your elbows are bent at 90-degree angles again, as you inhale. Repeat.

THRUSTERS

Stand with your feet shoulder-width apart while holding a dumbbell in each hand above your shoulders (your palms should be facing your ears). Keep your back flat and your knees behind your toes as you squat down until your thighs are parallel to the floor. Push through your heels as you return to a standing position while pushing the dumbbells overhead until your arms are fully extended. Return to the starting position. Repeat.

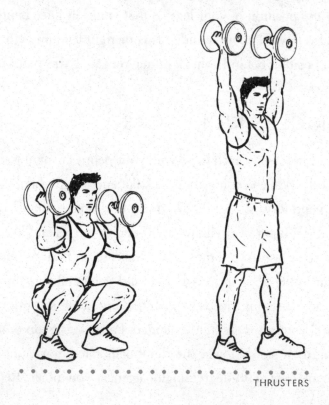

THRUSTERS

KNEE RAISES

Using a Captain's Chair or similar apparatus, place your fore-arms against the pads or bars and grip the handles or bars. Push yourself up so that your elbows are bent at 90-degree angles and your upper arms are in a straight line with the sides of your torso. Keep your torso straight and your head in line with your spine; press your lower back into the apparatus's pad if there is one. Start with your legs extended toward the floor. As you exhale, bend your knees and lift your legs up in a smooth, arc-like motion until your thighs are parallel to the floor. Gently lower them toward the floor again as you inhale. (Don't swing your legs up and down to create momentum; this should be performed in a smooth, controlled movement.) Repeat.

BACK EXTENSIONS

Stand with your hips and upper thighs against a hyperextension bench and anchor your ankles under or against the footpads. You should be able to bend freely from the waist. Start with your body in a straight line (from head to heel) with your arms crossed against your chest or behind your head. Slowly bend forward as far as you can without rounding your back, while tightening your ab and back muscles. Hold the lower position for a count, then slowly raise yourself back up to a straight line (don't arch your back at the top). Repeat.

INCLINE SIT-UPS

Lie back on an incline board that's set at an angle that's comfortable for you. Hook your feet under the pad to anchor yourself. Keep your knees slightly bent and your hands crossed over your chest or behind your ears. Slowly curl your body upward until your elbows touch your knees. Then slowly descend back down. (Keep the movements up and down slow, smooth, and controlled.) Repeat.

STRAIGHT BAR PULLDOWNS

Stand facing a cable station with your feet shoulder-width apart. Keep your lower back straight and your abs engaged as you grab a pulldown bar with a wide grip. While keeping a slight bend in your elbows, pull the bar straight down to your hips. Pause then slowly return to the start of the movement, without letting the weight rest against the stack. Repeat.

WALKOUTS

Stand with your legs fully extended, then bend from the hips and put your palms flat on the floor. Keep your legs straight as you lean forward and walk your hands as far forward as you can (don't let your hips sag!) until you're in a high plank position. Then, walk your feet to your hands by taking small steps. Repeat.

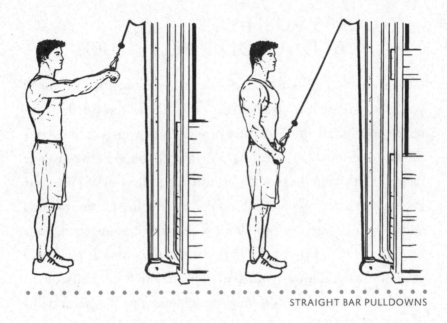

STRAIGHT BAR PULLDOWNS

PISTOL SQUATS

Stand with your feet hip-width apart and your hands by your sides. Lift your left foot and extend your left leg out in front of you as you raise both arms in front of you (to shoulder level). In a controlled movement, bend your right knee and lower your body toward the floor, pushing your hips back as if you were going to sit. Stop when your right thigh is parallel to the floor, pause for a moment, then rise, pushing through your right heel as you straighten your right leg and lower your arms to your sides again. Repeat for the desired number of reps. Switch sides. (Note: if this move is too difficult, you can hold onto a chair, bench, or TRX strap to help you with balance as you do this.)

TRICEPS PUSH-UPS
(A.K.A. DIAMOND PUSH-UPS)

Get down on the floor on all fours with your hands in front of you, shoulder-width apart. Bring your hands toward the center of your chest until the tips of your index fingers and your thumbs are touching, creating a diamond shape between your hands. With your fingers facing forward, lift yourself off your knees so that your body is in a straight line with only your hands and toes in contact with the floor. Keep your abs engaged, your back straight, and your head in line with your spine as you bend your elbows and lower your body toward the floor. Pause, then return to the starting position by straightening your arms and lifting your body. Repeat.

L-SIT

Position yourself between parallel bars and hold the bars with a neutral grip. Push your body off the ground, straightening your elbows as if you were at the top of a dip exercise. Keep your shoulders down, lock your knees, and hold your legs closely together as you raise them so your body is at a 90-degree angle from your legs to your torso. Your legs should be parallel to the floor. Hold this position for the desired duration.

APPENDIX B

RECIPES

HERE ARE SOME SERIOUSLY TASTY, NUTRIENT-PACKED RECIPES TO help you power up your energy while you're working to transform your body.

PROTEIN PANCAKES

1 SERVING

¼ cup raw oats
¼ cup cottage cheese
1 tablespoon chia seeds
½ scoop protein powder
½ cup egg whites
1 tablespoon coconut oil

Place all the ingredients in a blender and pulse until a batter forms. Melt 1 tablespoon coconut oil in a pan over medium heat and add the batter to form two or three pancakes. Cook them until bubbles have formed on the surface and the edges start to brown, then flip the pancakes over and cook on the other side. Serve with nuts, nut butter, and/or fruit.

BUTTERNUT SQUASH PANCAKES

1 cup cooked butternut squash (canned)
$^2/_3$ cup oats
2 medium eggs
½ teaspoon baking powder
1 tablespoon maple syrup
½ teaspoon ground cinnamon
¼ teaspoon sea salt
1 tablespoon coconut oil, plus more as needed
1 cup coconut Greek yogurt or skyr
Berries

Place the butternut squash, oats, eggs, baking powder, maple syrup, cinnamon, and salt in a blender and pulse until smooth. Heat 1 tablespoon coconut oil in a pan over medium heat. Drop scoops of the batter into the pan to make 2-inch pancakes. Cook for 2 to 3 minutes until bubbles have formed on the surface, then flip the pancakes over and cook the other side until the center is set. Remove from the heat while you cook the rest of the pancakes, adding more coconut oil as needed. Serve the pancakes with a large spoonful of yogurt and berries.

OMELET MUFFINS

4 SERVINGS

Butter
8 eggs
8 ounces cooked ham or turkey bacon, crumbled
1 cup diced red bell pepper
1 cup diced onion
¼ teaspoon salt
⅛ teaspoon ground black pepper
2 tablespoons water

Preheat the oven to 350°F. Lightly grease eight muffin cups with butter. In a large bowl, beat the eggs, then add the ham or turkey bacon, bell pepper, onion, salt, pepper, and water, mixing thoroughly. Pour the mixture evenly into the muffin cups. Bake until the omelet muffins are set in the middle, approximately 17 to 20 minutes.

CHIA PUDDING

2 SERVINGS

6 tablespoons chia seeds
2 cups unsweetened coconut, almond, or cashew milk
½ teaspoon vanilla extract
½ to 1 scoop protein powder (optional)
Berries, for serving

In a bowl or Mason jar, mix together the chia seeds, milk, vanilla, and protein powder (if using) until the ingredients are well combined. Let the mixture sit for 5 minutes, then stir it again to break up any clumps of chia seeds. Cover the mixture (or put the lid on the jar) and refrigerate it for 1 to 2 hours or overnight. It will be ready to eat when it's thick, not liquidy; if it's still runny after the designated refrigeration time, add more chia seeds, stir the mixture, and refrigerate it for another 30 minutes. To serve it, divide the mixture between two bowls and top them with berries.

MORNING PARFAIT

4 SERVINGS

1½ cups cooked quinoa
2 tablespoons chia seeds
½ cup raw almonds, chopped
2 cups Greek yogurt (plain or vanilla)
1 cup sliced strawberries
1 cup blueberries

Mix the quinoa, chia seeds, and almonds. Place ¼ cup yogurt in the base of each of four glasses or jars, then evenly distribute the quinoa mixture between the parfait vessels. Top each quinoa mixture with ¼ cup strawberries, followed by another ¼ cup yogurt, followed by ¼ cup blueberries. Cover the parfaits and refrigerate them overnight or until ready to serve.

ROASTED NECTARINES

4 SERVINGS

4 nectarines (or peaches), sliced
2 apricots, sliced
1 tablespoon coconut oil
1 tablespoon ground cinnamon

Preheat the oven to 400°F. In a large bowl, mix the fruits with the coconut oil and ground cinnamon. When the oven is ready, transfer the fruits to a nonstick baking pan and roast until soft and caramelized, about 20 to 25 minutes. Remove from the oven. Serve when warm or cool.

HUEVOS RANCHEROS

2 SERVINGS

2 large tomatoes, cored and chopped
½ small red onion, chopped
½ red bell pepper, chopped
1 tablespoon extra-virgin olive oil
1 small lime
Salt and pepper, to taste
1 tablespoon grapeseed oil
2 cloves garlic, minced
1 (15.5-ounce) can black beans, drained and rinsed
¼ cup water
¼ teaspoon ground coriander seed
2 (6-inch) corn tortillas
2 extra-large eggs
½ avocado, sliced

Mix the tomatoes, onion, and bell pepper with the olive oil and a little lime juice; season the mixture with salt and pepper and set aside. Add the grapeseed oil to a pan and sauté the garlic over moderate heat (don't let it change color), then add the black beans. Use a fork to smash the

continued

beans, adding ¼ cup water, a pinch of salt, and the coriander; when the mixture has thickened and is heated through, remove it from the heat. In a large skillet, toast the tortillas on both sides, then put them on plates and top them with the smashed black beans. Meanwhile, poach or fry the eggs. When the eggs are cooked, place them on top of the black beans. Serve with the tomato mixture and avocado slices.

GREEN JUICE

1 SERVING

1 kiwi, peeled
1 generous handful organic spinach leaves
1 cup coconut water
1 teaspoon chia seeds
Juice from ¼ lemon

Place all the ingredients in blender and blend until the drink is the desired texture. Drink immediately or chill it in the refrigerator until you're ready to consume it.

LENTIL SOUP

4 SERVINGS

1 tablespoon grapeseed oil
1 large onion, chopped
1 garlic clove, minced
1 cup chopped carrots
1 cup diced red bell pepper
2 cups low-sodium chicken or vegetable broth
1 cup dried lentils, rinsed
2 cups water
1 cup shredded spinach leaves (tough stems removed)
1 (14.5-ounce) can fire-roasted diced tomatoes, drained
½ teaspoon ground cumin
¼ teaspoon salt
Freshly ground pepper to taste

In a large pot, heat the grapeseed oil over medium heat. Sauté the onion, garlic, carrots, and pepper until soft, about 5–7 minutes. Add the broth, lentils, and water and bring to a boil. Reduce heat and let it simmer, covered, until the lentils are tender, about 45 minutes. Add spinach, tomatoes, cumin, salt, and pepper and cook, stirring occasionally, until the spinach softens, about 5 minutes. Adjust seasonings to taste, and serve.

VEGGIE FRITTATA

8 SERVINGS

1 tablespoon grapeseed oil
2 cloves garlic, minced
3 scallions, chopped
3 large zucchini, sliced
1 eggplant (unpeeled), sliced and chopped
½ lb. mushrooms, sliced
6 eggs
1 teaspoon Italian seasoning
1 teaspoon salt
½ teaspoon freshly ground pepper

Preheat the oven to 350°F. Heat the grapeseed oil in a large skillet over medium heat and sauté the garlic until soft, then add the veggies. Sauté the veggies, while stirring and turning them occasionally, for about 7 minutes (until they are soft but not mushy). Meanwhile, beat the eggs until they're frothy and add the seasonings. Place the vegetables in a rectangular baking dish, then pour the beaten eggs over them. Bake for 40 minutes, until the eggs have set and the top is slightly brown. Cut into servings and enjoy!

TURKEY CHILI

7 SERVINGS

1 tablespoon grapeseed oil
1 small onion, chopped
2 garlic cloves, minced
1½ lbs. lean ground turkey
1 teaspoon chili powder
½ tablespoon cumin
½ tablespoon oregano
1 teaspoon red pepper flakes
2 (15.5-ounce) cans of cannellini beans, rinsed
    and drained
1 cup chicken broth
Salt and pepper, to taste
½ red onion, chopped (optional)
Fresh cilantro (optional)

Heat the grapeseed oil in a large pot over medium heat. Add the onions and garlic and sauté until soft, about 5 minutes. Add the ground turkey and cook it until it's white, breaking up clumps with a fork. Stir in the chili powder, cumin, oregano, and red pepper flakes and cook for 2 minutes. Add

continued

the beans and broth and cook uncovered for 10 minutes. Lower the heat, cover the pot, and let the chili simmer for another 30 to 45 minutes, stirring occasionally. Add salt and pepper, to taste. Serve with chopped red onion and fresh cilantro, if desired.

LENTIL SALAD

4 Servings

2½ cups cooked lentils (cooled)
½ cup chopped red bell pepper
½ red onion, diced
1 cup chopped sugar snap peas
½ cup chopped carrots

For the dressing:
4 tablespoons extra-virgin olive oil
4 tablespoons balsamic vinegar
2 teaspoons Dijon mustard
1 teaspoon minced garlic
Salt and pepper, to taste

In a large bowl, mix the first five ingredients together. Whisk the ingredients for the dressing together, then pour it over the lentil mixture. Stir well to combine all the ingredients and the dressing. Serve.

SELECTED BIBLIOGRAPHY

Bolonchuk, W. W., et al. "Association of Dominant Somatotype of Men with Body Structure, Function During Exercise, and Nutritional Assessment." *American Journal of Human Biology* 12, no. 2 (March 2000): 167–180. https://www.ncbi.nlm.nih.gov /pubmed/11534013.

Burg, M. M., et al. "Does Stress Result in You Exercising Less? Or Does Exercising Result in You Being Less Stressed? Or Is It Both?" *Annals of Behavioral Medicine* 51, no. 6 (December 2017): 799–809. https://www.ncbi.nlm.nih.gov/pmc/articles /PMC5597451/.

Cárdenas-Fernández, V., et al. "Somatotype and Body Composition in Young Soccer Players According to the Playing Position and Sport Success." *Journal of Strength and Conditioning Research* (July 2017). https://www.ncbi.nlm.nih.gov/pubmed/28723818.

Carter, J. E. L. "The Heath-Carter Anthropomorphic Somatotype Instruction Manual." March 2002. http://www.somatotype.org /Heath-CarterManual.pdf.

Carvajal, W., et al. "Body Type and Performance of Elite Cuban Baseball Players." *MEDICC Review* 11, no. 2 (April 2009): 15–20. https://www.ncbi.nlm.nih.gov/pubmed/21483313.

Chaouachi, M., et al. "Effects of Dominant Somatotype on Aerobic Capacity Trainability." *British Journal of Sports Medicine* 39, no. 12 (December 2005): 954–959. https://www.ncbi.nlm.nih.gov/pmc/articles/PMC1725084/.

"Early Release of Selected Estimates Based on Data from the National Health Interview Survey, 2016." Centers for Disease Control and Prevention (May 2017). https://www.cdc.gov/nchs/data/nhis/earlyrelease/Earlyrelease201705_07.pdf.

Fernández-López, J. R., et al. "The Effect of Morphological and Functional Variables on Ranking Position of Professional Junior Basque Surfers." *European Journal of Sport Science* 13, no. 5 (2013): 461–467. https://www.ncbi.nlm.nih.gov/pubmed/24050462.

Fitzgerald, M. *How Bad Do You Want It? Mastering the Psychology of Mind over Muscle.* Boulder, CO: Velo, 2015.

Gomez-Ezeiza, J., et al. "Anthropometric Characteristics of Top-Class Olympic Race Walkers." *Journal of Sports Medicine and Physical Fitness* (April 20, 2018). https://www.ncbi.nlm.nih.gov/pubmed/29687690.

Gutnik, B., et al. "Body Physique and Dominant Somatotype in Elite and Low-Profile Athletes with Different Specializations." *Medicina* 51, no. 4 (2015): 247–252. https://www.ncbi.nlm.nih.gov/pubmed/26424190.

Karageorghis, C. I., and P. C. Terry. *Inside Sport Psychology.* Champaign, IL: Human Kinetics, 2011.

Katzmarzyk, P. T., et al. "Familial Resemblance for Physique: Heritabilities for Somatotype Components." *Annals of Human Biology* 27, no. 5 (2000): 467–477. https://www.ncbi.nlm.nih.gov/pubmed/11023117.

Knowles, O. E., et al. "Inadequate Sleep and Muscle Strength: Implications for Resistance Training." *Journal of Science and Medicine in Sport* 21, no. 9 (September 2018): 959–968. https://www.ncbi.nlm.nih.gov/pubmed/29422383.

La Bounty, P. M., et al. "International Society of Sports Nutrition Position Stand: Meal Frequency." *Journal of the International Society of Sports Nutrition* 8, no. 4 (2011). https://jissn.biomedcentral.com/articles/10.1186/1550-2783-8-4.

Levine, J. A., et al. "Energy Expenditure of Nonexercise Activity." *American Journal of Clinical Nutrition* 72, no. 6 (December 2000): 1451–1454. https://www.ncbi.nlm.nih.gov/pubmed/11101470.

Levine, J. A., et al. "Role of Nonexercise Activity Thermogenesis in Resistance to Fat Gain in Humans." *Science* 283, no. 5399 (January 1999): 212–214. https://www.ncbi.nlm.nih.gov/pubmed/9880251.

Lindsay, E. "Sleep Restriction Decreases the Physical Activity of Adults at Risk for Type 2 Diabetes." *Sleep* 35, no. 7 (July 2012): 977–984. https://www.ncbi.nlm .nih.gov/pmc/articles/PMC3369233/.

Martínez, J. G., et al. "Position-Specific Anthropometry and Throwing Velocity of Elite Female Water Polo Players." *Journal of Strength and Conditioning Research* 29, no. 2 (February 2015): 472–477. https://www.ncbi.nlm.nih.gov /pubmed/25627450.

Martínez-Rodríguez, A., et al. "Body Composition Assessment of Paddle and Tennis Adult Male Players." *Nutrición Hospitalaria* 31, no. 3 (September 2014): 1294–1301. https://www.ncbi.nlm.nih.gov/pubmed/25726225.

Martin-Matillas, M., et al. "Anthropometric, Body Composition and Somatotype Characteristics of Elite Female Volleyball Players from the Highest Spanish League." *Journal of Sports Sciences* 32, no. 2 (2014): 137–148. https://www .ncbi.nlm.nih.gov/pubmed/23879184.

Mifflin, M. D., et al. "A New Predictive Equation for Resting Energy Expenditure in Healthy Individuals." *American Journal of Clinical Nutrition* 51, no. 2 (1990): 241–247. https://www.ncbi.nlm.nih.gov/pubmed/2305711.

Moyer, A. E., et al. "Stress-Induced Cortisol Response and Fat Distribution in Women." *Obesity Research* 2, no. 3 (May 1994): 255–262. https://www.ncbi .nlm.nih.gov/pubmed/16353426.

Ozimek, M., et al. "Somatic Profile of the Elite Boulderers in Poland." *Journal of Strength and Conditioning Research* 31, no. 4 (April 2017): 963–970. https:// www.ncbi.nlm.nih.gov/pubmed/28328714.

Park, H. K., et al. "Physiology of Leptin: Energy Homeostasis, Neuroendocrine Function and Metabolism." *Metabolism* 64, no. 1 (January 2015): 24–34. https:// www.sciencedirect.com/science/article/pii/S0026049514002418.

Plante, T. G. "Could the Perception of Fitness Account for Many of the Mental and Physical Health Benefits of Exercise?" *Advances in Mind-Body Medicine* 15, no. 4 (Fall 1999): 291–295. https://www.ncbi.nlm.nih.gov/pubmed/10555401.

Sánchez-Muñoz, C., et al. "World and Olympic Mountain Bike Champions' Anthropometry, Body Composition and Somatotype." *Journal of Sports Medicine and Physical Fitness* 58, no. 6 (June 2018): 843–851. https://www.ncbi.nlm.nih .gov/pubmed/28462576.

Schroeder, E. T., et al. "Are Acute Post-Resistance Exercise Increases in Testosterone, Growth Hormone, and IGF-1 Necessary to Stimulate Skeletal Muscle Anabolism and Hypertrophy?" *Medicine and Science in Sports and Exercise* 45, no. 11 (2013): 2044–2051. https://www.researchgate.net/publication/258055839_Are_Acute

_Post-Resistance_Exercise_Increases_in_Testosterone_Growth_Hormone_and_ IGF-1_Necessary_to_Stimulate_Skeletal_Muscle_Anabolism_and_Hypertrophy.

Shariat, A., et al. "Kinanthropometric Attributes of Elite Male Judo, Karate and Taekwondo Athletes." *Revista Brasileira de Medicina do Esporte* 23, no 4 (July–August 2017). http://www.scielo.br/scielo.php?pid=S1517-86922017 000400260&script=sci_arttext.

Silva, D. A., et al. "Anthropometric Profiles of Elite Older Triathletes in the Ironman Brazil Compared with Those of Young Portuguese Triathletes and Older Brazilians." *Journal of Sports Sciences* 30, no. 5 (2012): 479–484. https://www.ncbi .nlm.nih.gov/pubmed/22260093.

Singh, K., et al. "Study of Body Composition and Somatotyping Among the Throwers." *International Journal of Physical Education, Sports and Health* 4, no. 4 (2017): 221–225. https://pdfs.semanticscholar.org/e8cf/b136595f2dda4a339 fe401dd684f8b381a34.pdf.

Slusher, A. L., et al. "Impact of High Intensity Interval Exercise on Executive Function and Brain Derived Neurotrophic Factor in Healthy College Aged Males." *Physiology and Behavior* 191 (July 2018): 116–122. https://www.ncbi.nlm.nih .gov/pubmed/29673858.

"Somatotype and Constitutional Psychology." *Wikipedia*, https://en.wikipedia.org /wiki/Somatotype_and_constitutional_psychology.

Vila, H., et al. "Anthropometric Profile, Vertical Jump, and Throwing Velocity in Elite Female Handball Players by Playing Positions." *Journal of Strength and Conditioning Research* 26, no. 8 (August 2012): 2146–2155. https://www.ncbi .nlm.nih.gov/pubmed/21997459.

Villablanca, P. A., et al. "Nonexercise Activity Thermogenesis in Obesity Management." *Mayo Clinic Proceedings* 90, no. 4 (April 2015): 509–519. https://www .ncbi.nlm.nih.gov/pubmed/25841254.

Wang, Q. P., et al. "Sucralose Promotes Food Intake Through NPY and a Neuronal Fasting Response." *Cell Metabolism* 24, no. 1 (July 2016): 75–90. https://www.cell.com/cell-metabolism/fulltext/S1550-4131(16)30296-0 ?_returnURL=https%3A%2F%2Flinkinghub.elsevier.com%2Fretrieve %2Fpii%2FS1550413116302960%3Fshowall%3Dtrue.

Wang, X., et al. "Sleep Quality Improved Following a Single Session of Moderate-Intensity Aerobic Exercise in Older Women: Results from a Pilot Study." *Journal of Sport and Health Science* 3, no. 4 (December 2014): 338–342. https://www .ncbi.nlm.nih.gov/pubmed/25685605.

ACKNOWLEDGMENTS

To Stacey Colino, the one and only: THANK YOU! Who knew Instagram messages worked for real?! Thank you for taking a chance on an Internet stranger and turning phone calls, celebrity magazine articles, and a book concept into reality. You helped me achieve my biggest goal and held my hand with patience along the way. Thank you from the bottom of my heart for making this happen.

To my brother, Dave: thank you for being my health role model and for teaching me so much throughout my life. To my amazing family, clients, and friends: you all have helped me in countless ways, and this book is a physical symbol of what we have built together. With all my heart, thank you! We did it, guys!

An extra-big thank you to my agent, Rick Broadhead, who championed this book from start to finish, and editor Dan Ambrosio, who was passionate about this subject from the get-go. Dan, your enthusiasm, support, and good cheer throughout the process helped make writing this book a labor of love for Stacey and me.

INDEX